Calm and Serene

CONQUERING ANXIETY WITH ESSENTIAL OIL

Rebecca Park Totilo

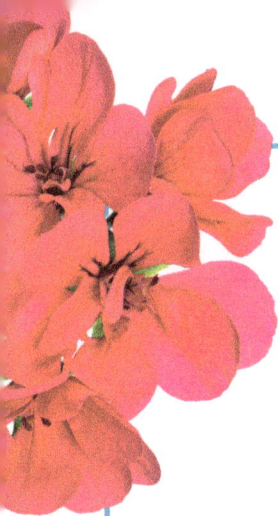

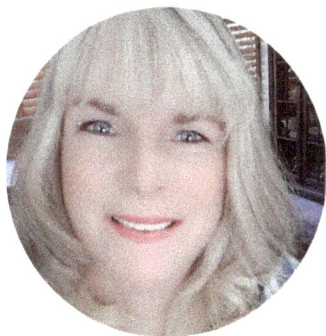

A Word from Rebecca

In the United States, 77% of people experience chronic or frequent stress-related symptoms. Of those, just over half report fatigue; another 44% report headaches; and just over 60% report muscle fatigue or stomach problems. Stress is a national epidemic, and there are no signs of it slowing down.

People are searching for new ways to cope. While most understand how our health and well-being depend on a balanced lifestyle, most of us continue to be driven by excessive pressures and expectations. Is it any wonder that stress and stress management has become such an integral part of modern living?

Fortunately, relief does not always need to come by prescription or cost you an arm and a leg. There is an answer for this epidemic which has been slowly gaining acceptance in the modern world: essential oils.

Essential oils are a natural, practical choice for stress relief due to their quick action without harmful side effects, and they can be used in many ways.

If you're unsure how to use your oils, read on to learn more about how stress affects your health and how to manage your stress levels better. With essential oils, you will learn how to relax your mind and body, allowing you to enjoy life more without the constant worry that stress brings.

Rebecca Park Totilo

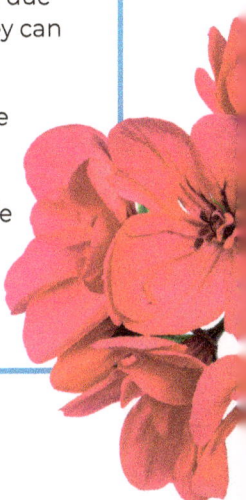

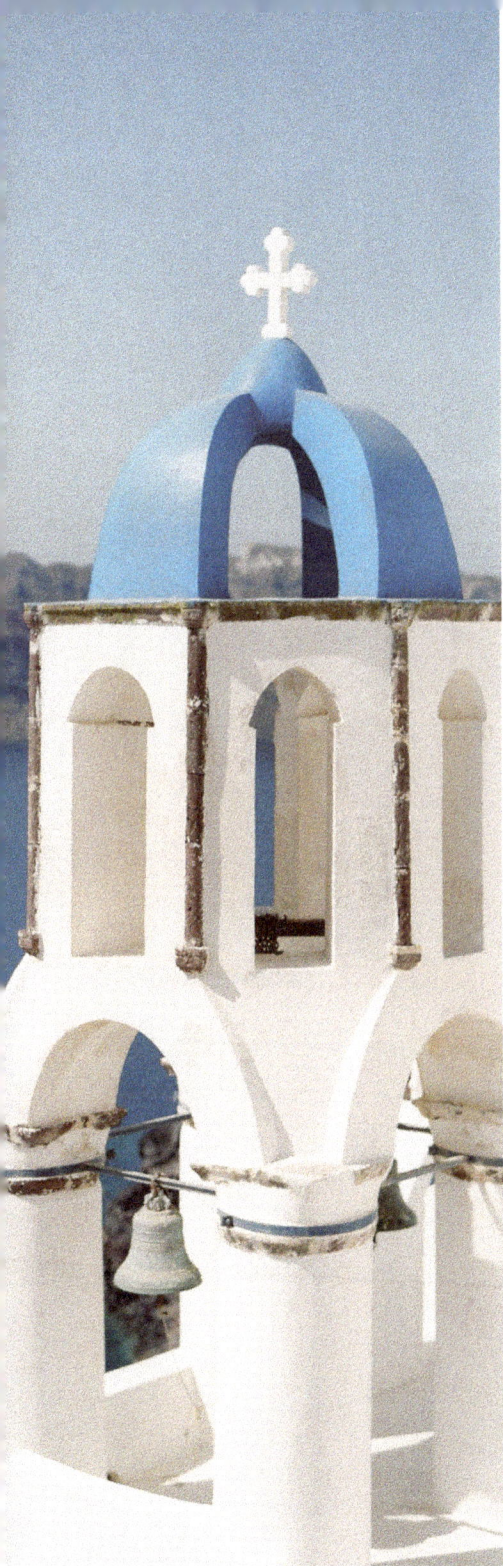

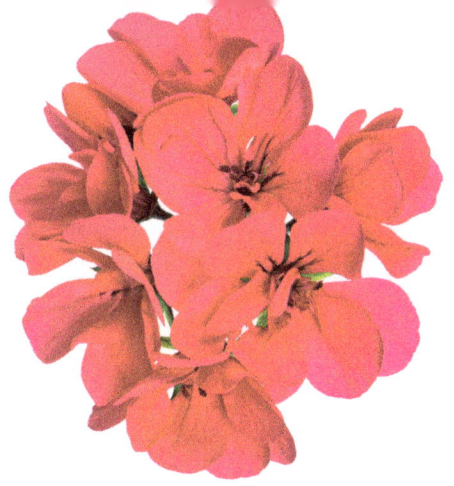

CONTENTS

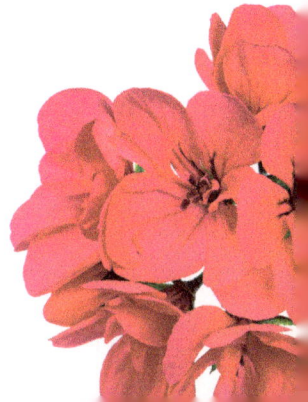

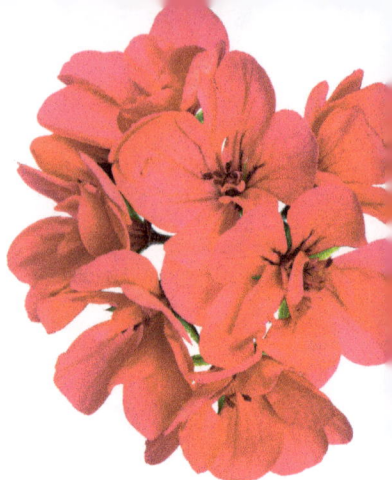

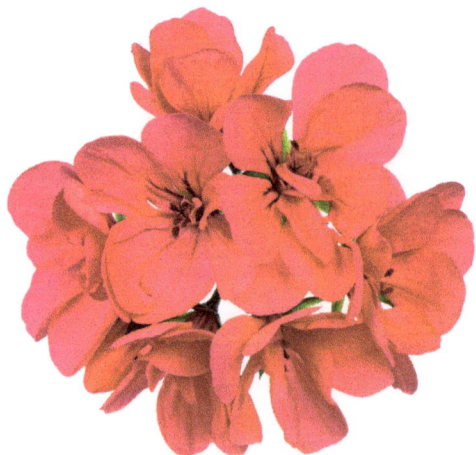

01/

INTRODUCTION TO CALM AND SERENE

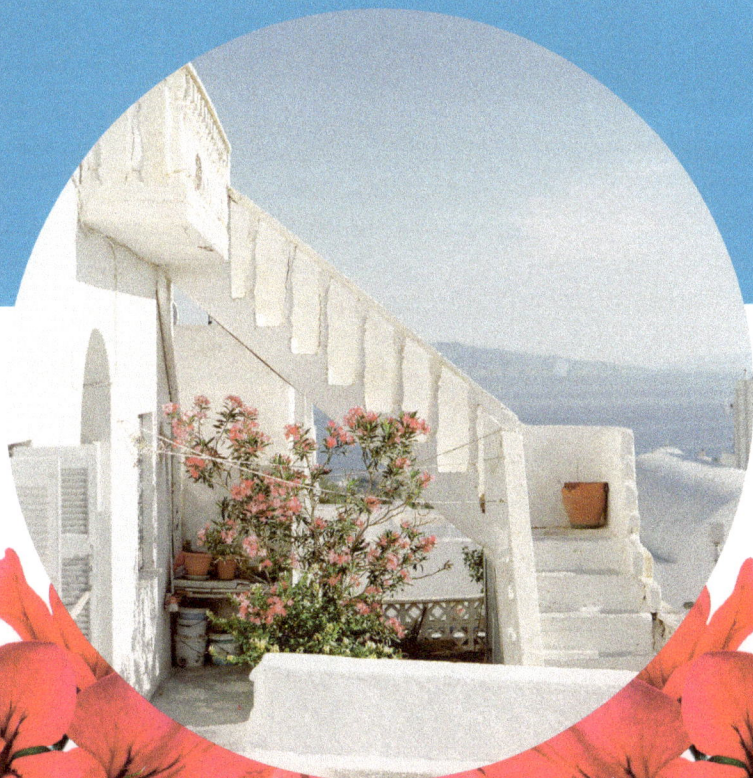

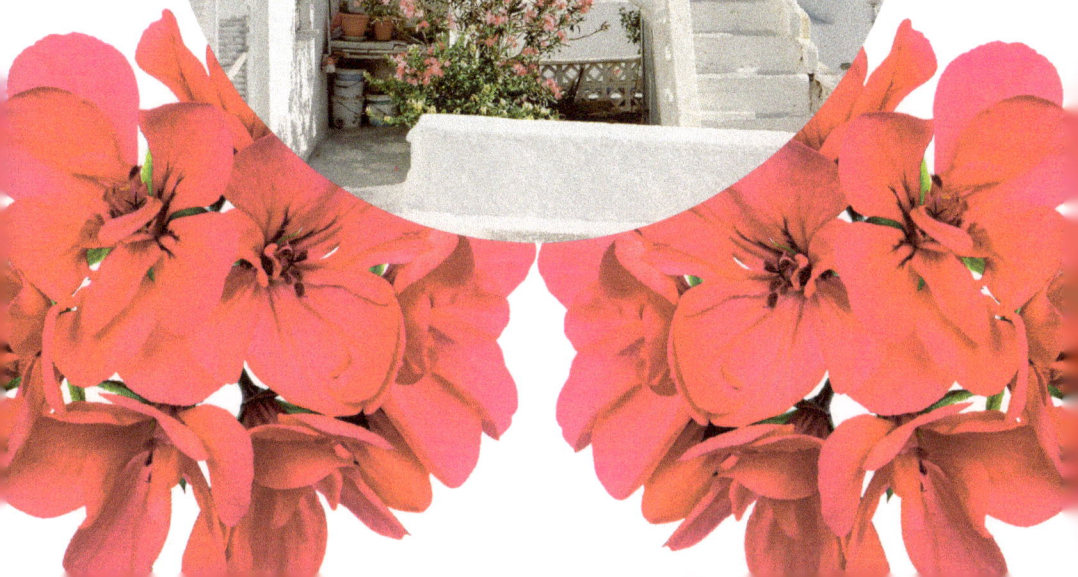

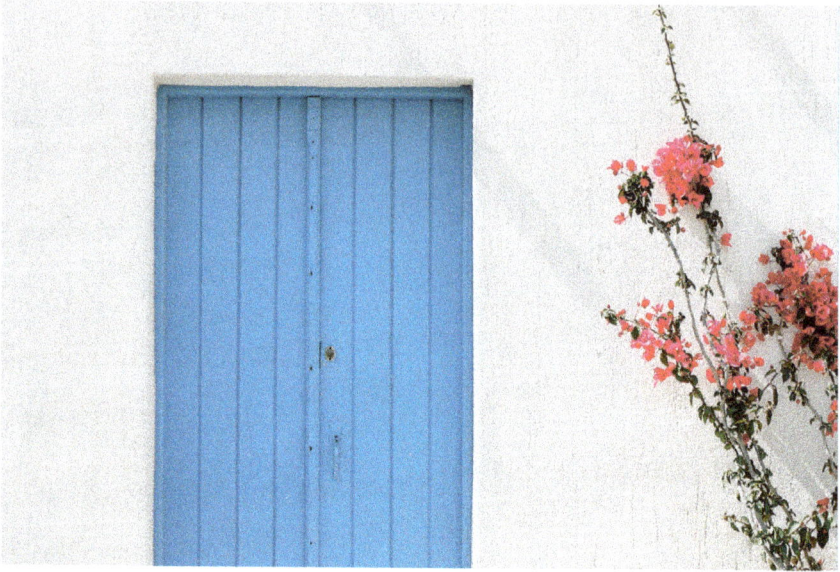

Most people regularly experience anxiety and worry, especially in stressful situations like passing a test, speaking in front of an audience, participating in a competitive sport, or attending a job interview. You may feel tense yet focused when experiencing this type of anxiety, which enables you to work more quickly or at your peak. Sometimes anxiety can get us to act, motivating us to do something about our situation. However, chronic anxiety can also eat away at our well-being, often leaving us feeling miserable, helpless, and stuck.

In this book, we will look at the tools, techniques, and essential oils that you can use in your everyday life to relieve you from anxiety. Overcoming anxiety can be a long journey, and I want to congratulate you for taking the first step to change your life with this book.

Self-care is an important part of your daily routine and should be planned into your schedule in order to reap all the benefits.

02 /

WHAT IS ANXIETY?

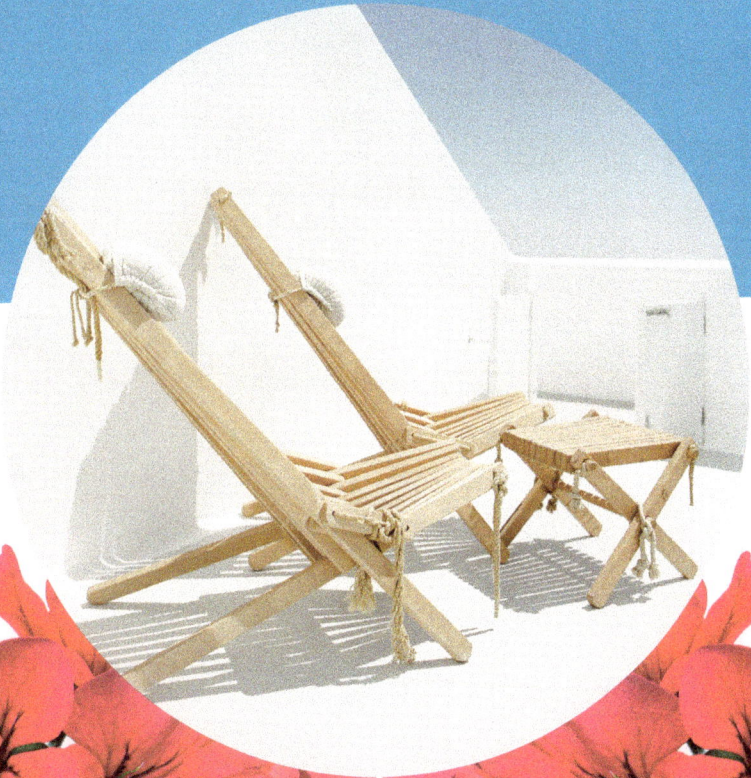

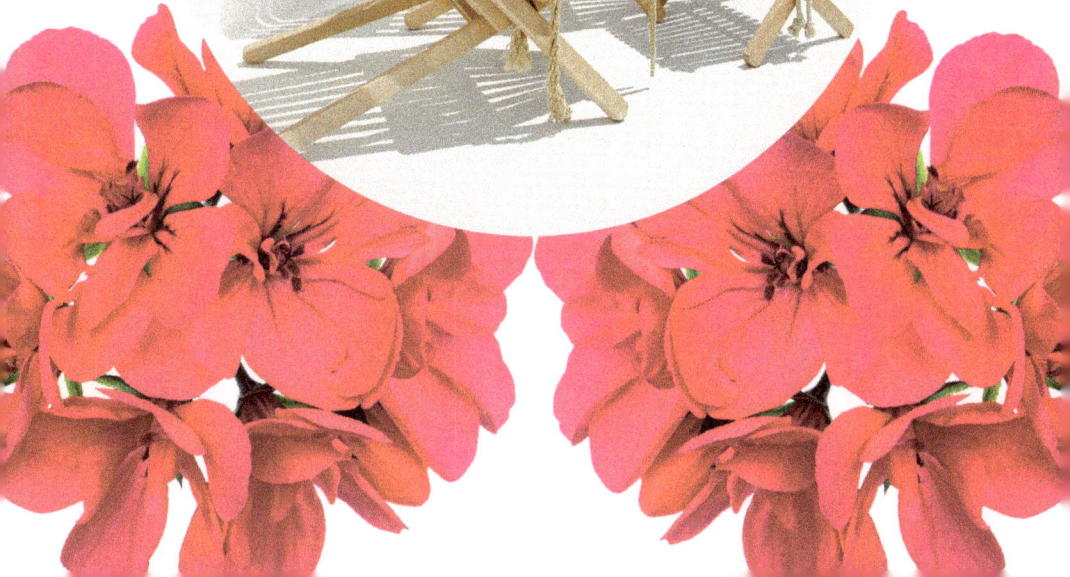

Anxiety is a common emotion when dealing with daily stresses and problems. But when these persistent, excessive, and irrational emotions affect a person's ability to function, anxiety becomes a disorder. Different types of anxiety disorders include phobias, panic and stress disorders, and obsessive-compulsive disorders.

When you're experiencing it, you may notice apprehension or a sense of foreboding, worry, and muscle tension. You may feel keyed up and on edge. You may detect that the bodily changes associated with anxiety are much less pronounced and dramatic than fear. Yet anxiety and worry can last much longer than fear, often ebbing and flowing for days, weeks, months, or even years. This is partly possible because anxiety tends to be fueled more by what your mind does than by real sources of danger or threat.

And as hard as it may be to experience anxiety, it's important to be mindful that you still need the capacity to experience anxiety. Why? Because it can help motivate you to get things done and keep you out of harm's way.

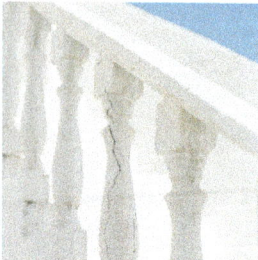

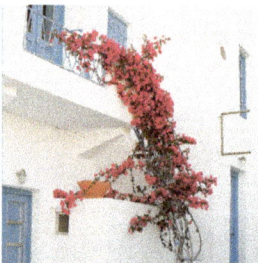

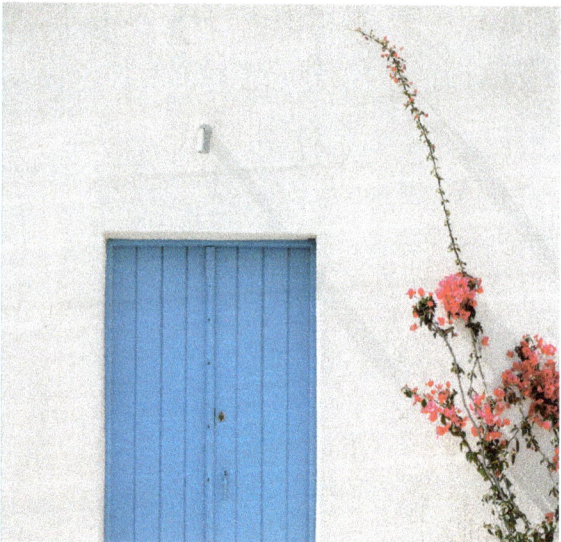

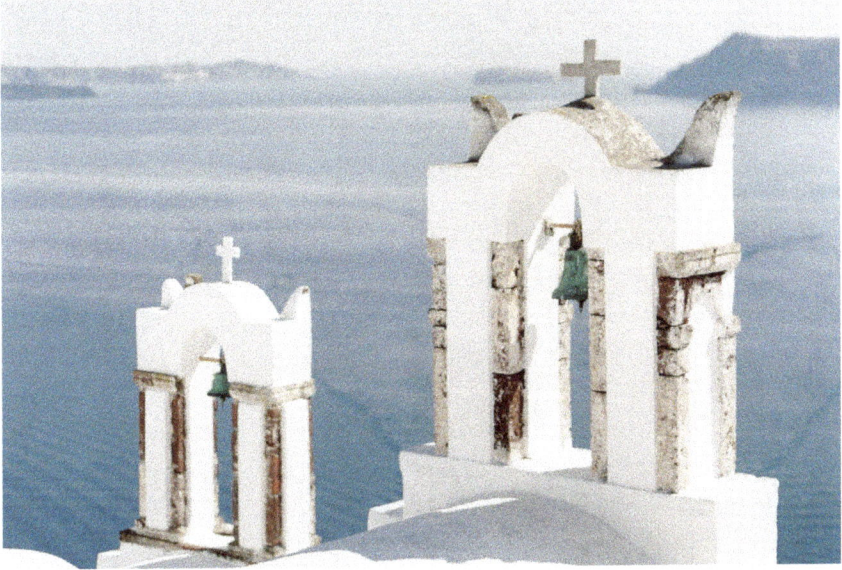

HOW DO YOU KNOW IF YOU ARE EXPERIENCING ANXIETY?

Some of the more common symptoms of anxiety include increased heart rate, palpitations, sweating, dizziness, headaches, upset stomach, shortness of breath, and difficulty concentrating.

Anxiety is a mental health condition, which means it's a condition that can affect the way you think, feel, and behave. Even though it's a "mental health" condition, anxiety can affect how you feel physically in your body and mind.

There are different types of anxiety, including generalized anxiety disorder, social anxiety, phobias, and panic disorder. It's common for people to experience more than one of these types of anxiety at the same time. Anxiety can also be present in conditions like depression, obsessive-compulsive disorder, and post-traumatic stress disorder.

Like all mental health conditions, anxiety is a medical condition. It can be treated, and without treatment, it can severely affect a person's life.

We have all felt anxious at some point in our lives—usually before important events such as going for a job interview, starting a new job, or speaking publicly for the first time. Anxiety becomes a problem if we feel it too intensely over small matters. If anxiety prevents us from leading an everyday life, professional help is needed.

For example, you may be anxious about your child's health, making mistakes at work, or the sales numbers for your business.

Some people struggle to pinpoint the causes of anxiety. If this is you, read on to get a clear idea of the cause of your anxiety. You should feel calmer after laying out your anxiety triggers in front of you and knowing how to address each one.

HOW DO YOU TURN OFF YOUR MIND AT NIGHT?

The racing thoughts that occupy your mind during the day don't automatically shut off because it's time to go to bed. So, to slow down and calm your mind at night, you should ensure you have time to relax without mental stimulation to ease into sleep.

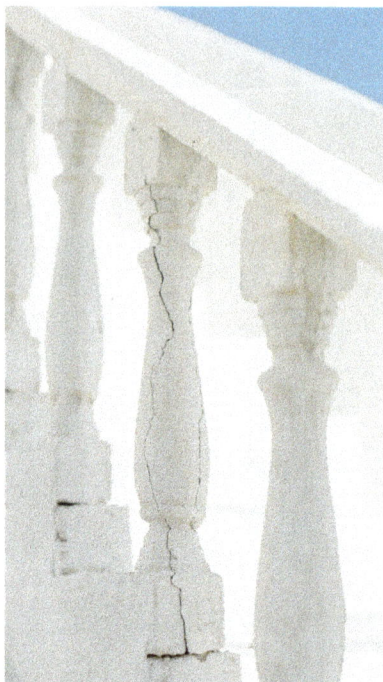

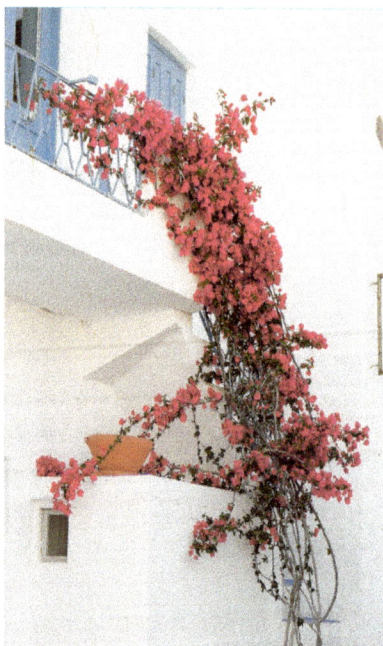

03

SYMPTOMS OF ANXIETY

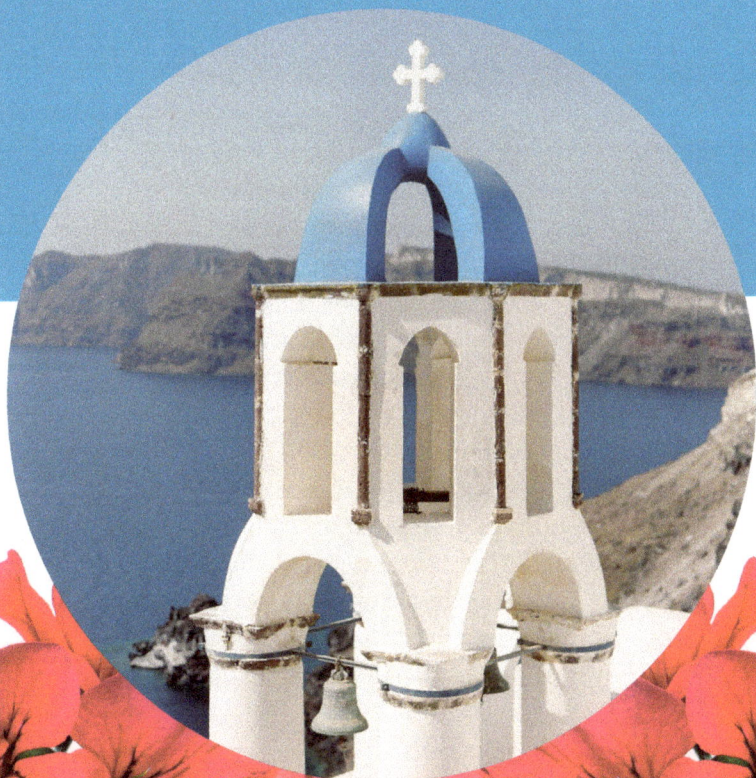

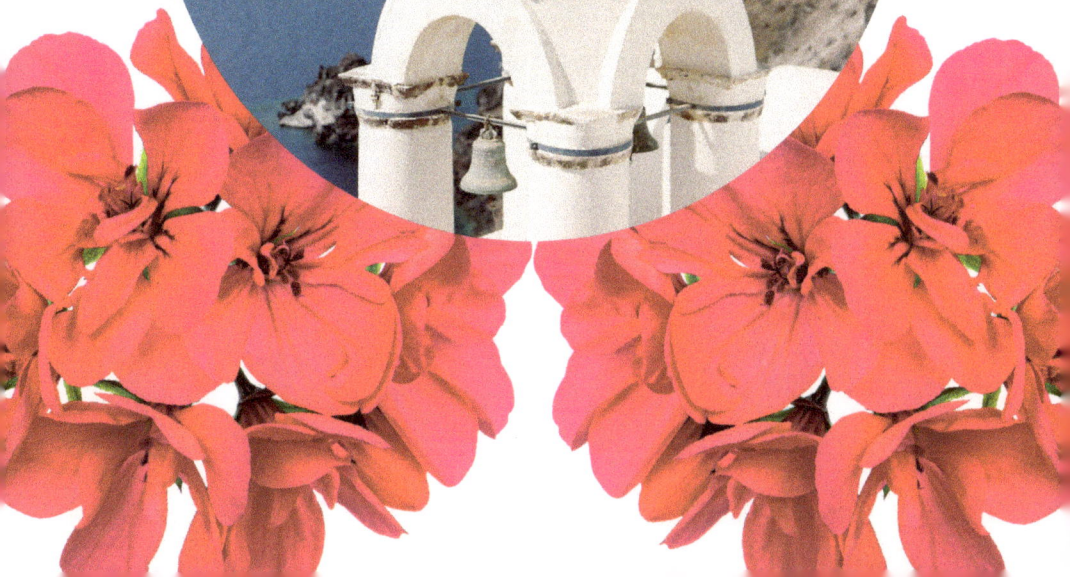

SYMPTOMS OF ANXIETY

Anxiety comes and goes, only lasting a short time for most people. Some moments of anxiety are briefer than others, lasting anywhere from a few minutes to a few days. But for some people, these anxiety feelings are more than passing worries or a stressful day at work.

- Nervousness, restlessness, or being tense
- Feelings of danger, panic, or dread
- Rapid heart rate - A racing heart beat is a common symptom associated with anxiety attacks. Most people will feel this in their chest rather than by actually testing their heart rate via a pulse point.
- Rapidly breathing, or hyperventilation - If you realize you are panting or taking rapid, shallows breaths, this can signify an anxiety attack. You may feel pressure or a weight on your chest or as if you cannot inhale to your full lung capacity.
- Tightness in the stomach - A feeling of a ball or fist in the pit of your gut can be a sign of an anxiety attack. This uncomfortable symptom of a panic attack is physically the same thing that happens in actual life-threatening situations, as fear provokes our bodies towards a fight-or-flight response to danger.
- Increased or heavy sweating
- Dizziness, tingling, changes in blood pressure, trembling, or muscle twitching - Many symptoms of an anxiety attack are due to an increase in blood pressure. As a result, you may experience dizziness or a tingling sensation in your arms, hands, and fingers.

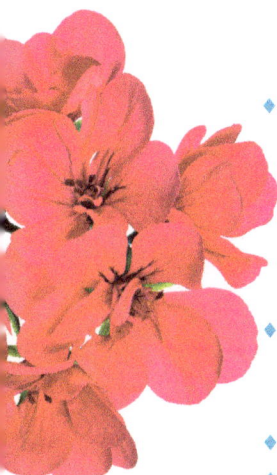

- Muscle tension, weakness, and lethargy - Muscular tightness in your neck, shoulders, and upper back can also be signs of having an anxiety attack. It's common for people having an anxiety attack to end up in the emergency room thinking they are having a heart attack.
- Difficulty focusing or thinking clearly about anything other than the thing you're worried about
- Insomnia
- Chills - Getting the chills, shivering, or the opposite, sweating in the palms of your hands, armpits, or arms are signs you may be having a panic attack.
- A strong desire to avoid the things that trigger your anxiety
- Performing certain behaviors over and over again
- Anxiety surrounding a particular life event or experience that has occurred in the past, especially indicative of post-traumatic stress disorder
- Feeling out of control - This is something that many people experience at the onset of an anxiety attack.

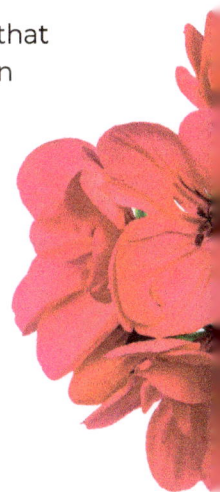

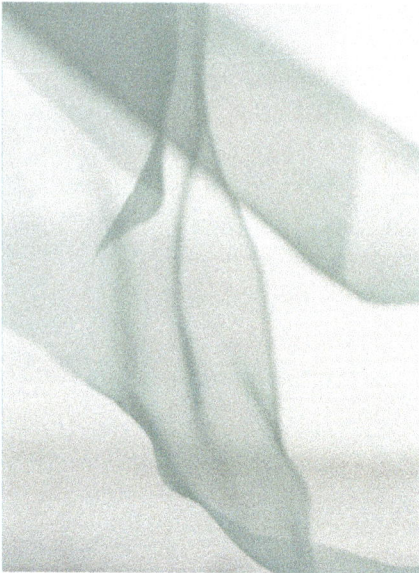

WHAT YOU CAN DO IF YOUR ANXIETY ESCALATES INTO A PANIC ATTACK

The most common signs of anxiety include racing thoughts, increased heart rate, fast breathing, stomach upset, shaking hands, sweating, and ruminating thoughts when one thought or worry keeps playing in your mind. If you begin to experience the signs of increased anxiety, you can use essential oils to help you to lower the anxiety before panic has a chance to set in. Other coping skills include deep breathing, exercising, and meditating, while using essential oils.

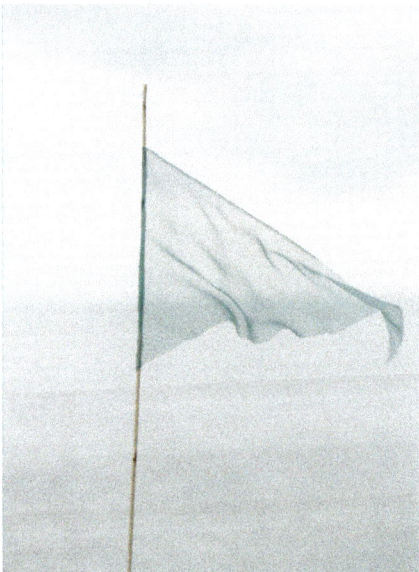

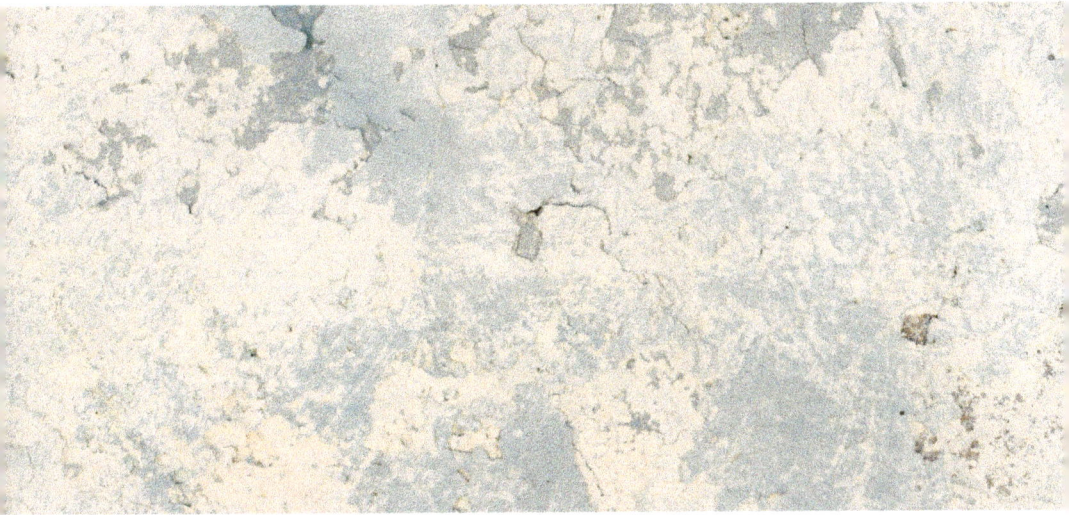

THE SIGNS OF ANXIETY

Excessive Worrying

According to the National Institute of Mental Health, individuals with anxiety disorders often worry excessively or have a sense of dread, usually lasting six months or longer. These anxious feelings can stem from school, the workplace, social interactions, personal relationships, health, or finances, to name a few causes.

In addition to breathing exercises using an essential oil, concentrate on your immediate surroundings. Identify five things that you can see, four things you can touch, three things you can hear, two things you can smell, and one thing you can taste.

Difficulties with Sleeping & Restlessness

It is very common for anxiety to keep people awake at night, especially the night before an event that is contributing to the fear and tension.

Fatigue

Even if the individual manages to fall asleep and get an adequate amount, someone who experiences anxiety may feel unsatisfied, experience fatigue throughout the day, or become tired.

Concentration Issues

Having difficulty concentrating is a common symptom of anxiety that can also be considered a side effect of worry or sleep problems.

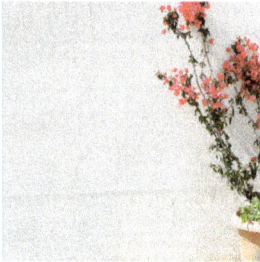

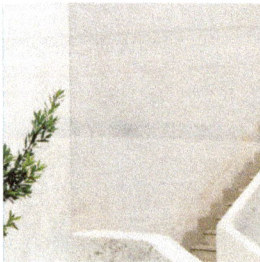

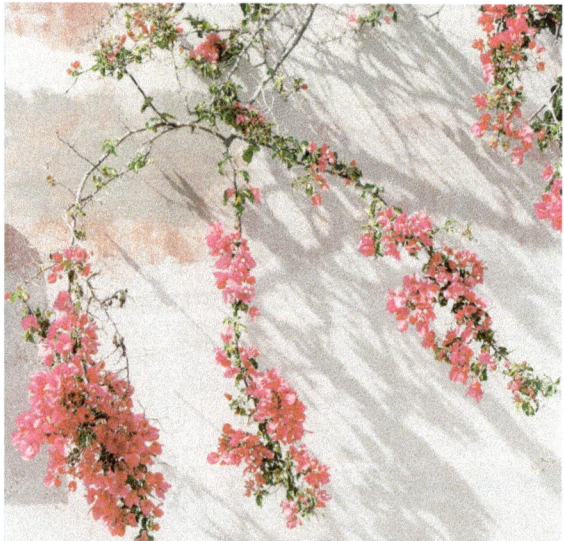

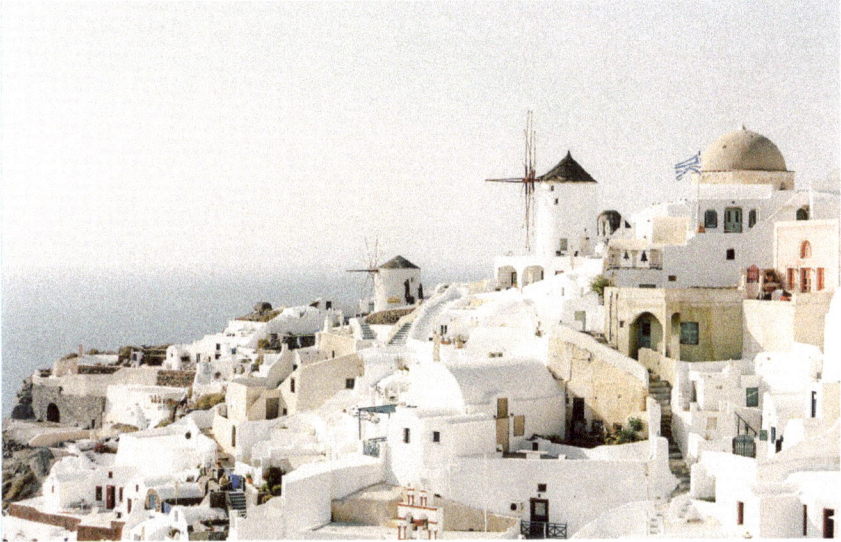

Increased Heart Rate & Palpitations

When faced with a situation that induces stress, a person may notice that their heart rate goes up or begins to feel irregular.

Sweating & Hot Flashes

An increase in body temperature often comes from increased heart rate and blood pressure.

Trembling & Shaking

The stress associated with anxiety can cause a person's limbs to shake uncontrollably, especially the hands.

> *Essential oils work in connection with the body. Therefore, paying attention to the oil's therapeutic effect is highly recommended.*

04/

TYPES OF ANXIETY

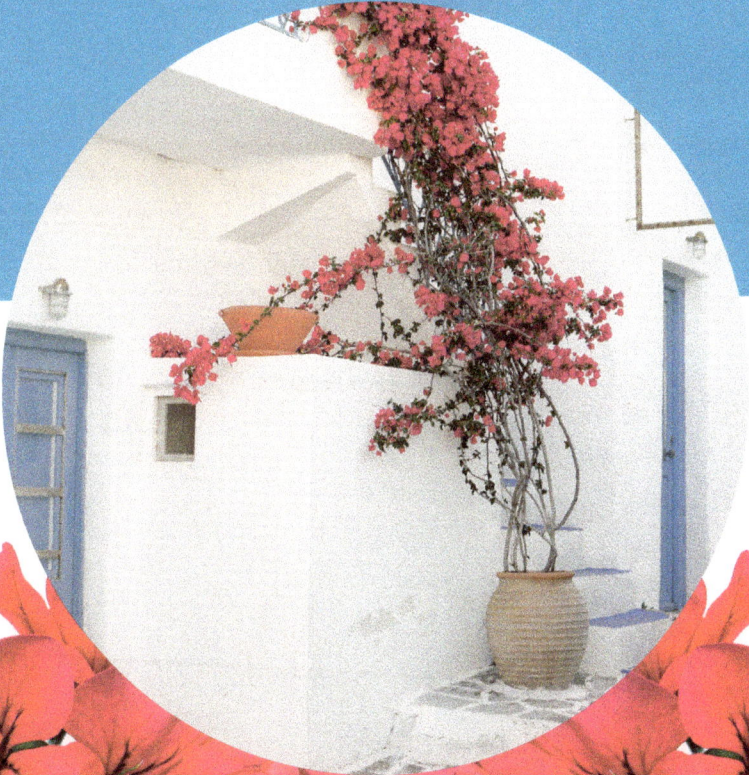

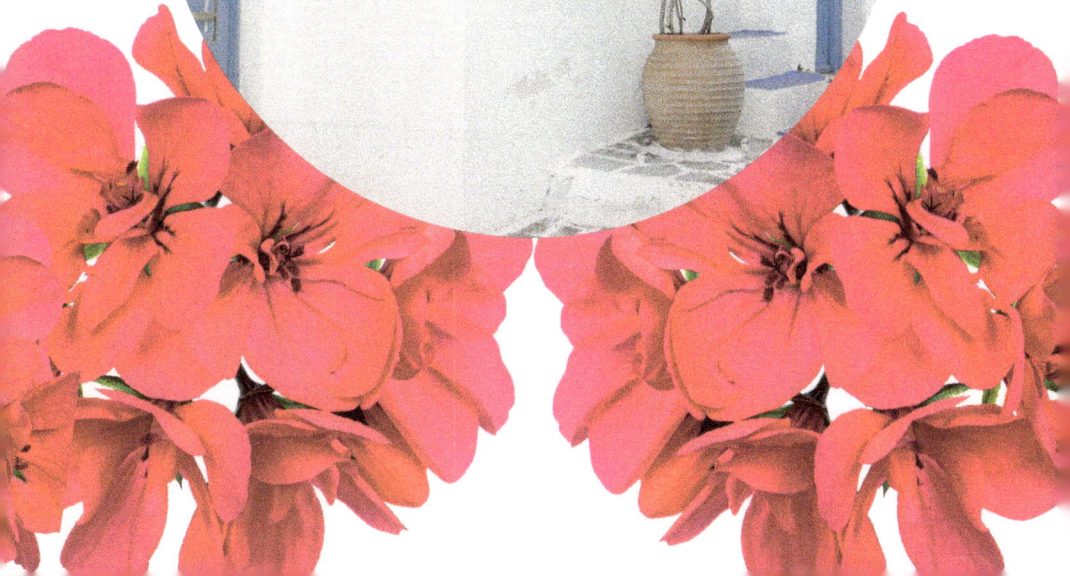

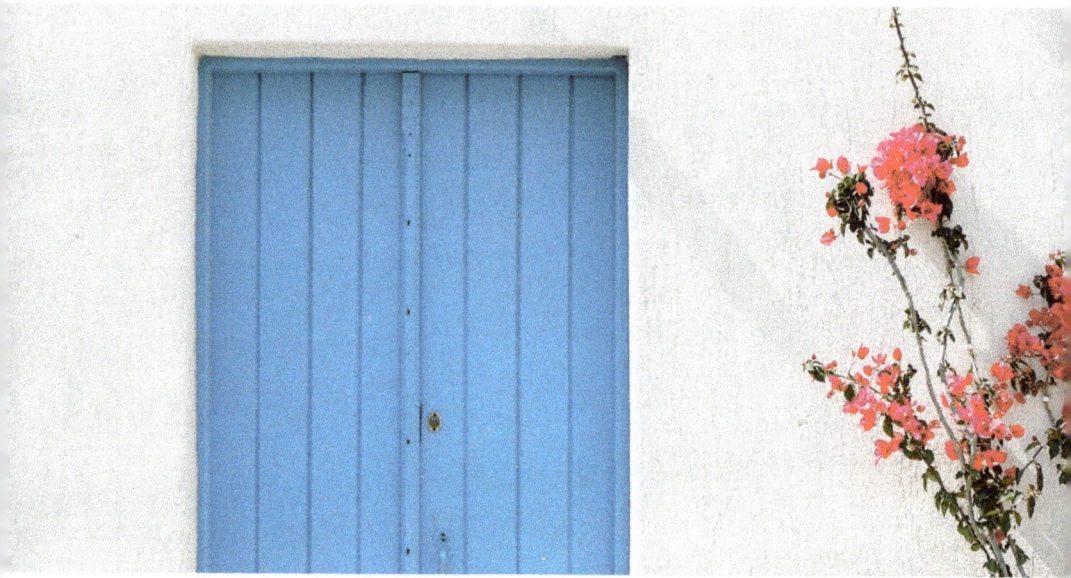

General Anxiety Disorder (GAD)

GAD, or general anxiety disorder, can eat away at a person's well-being, often leaving someone feeling miserable, helpless, and stuck. People with GAD always have strong, ongoing worry, not only during certain stressful circumstances, and the anxiety interferes with their daily life. They are concerned about various aspects of everyday life rather than simply one, such as work, health, family, or financial concerns. Even seemingly unimportant actions, like doing the dishes or running late for an appointment, can cause worry, leading to uncontrollable worries.

People with GAD have strong, ongoing worry, not only during certain stressful circumstances that interfere with their daily life.

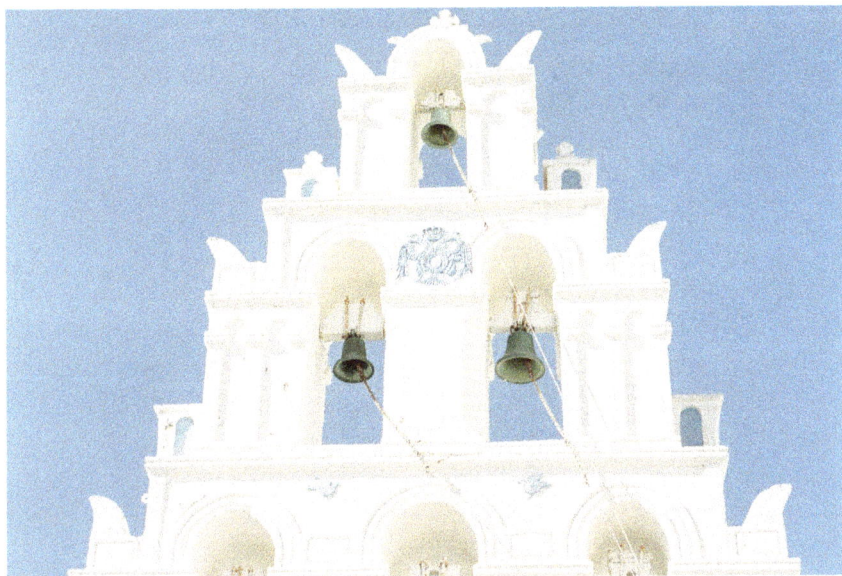

Obsessive-Compulsive Disorder (OCD)

Our behavior can sometimes be influenced by anxious thoughts that could be beneficial. For instance, you might check the oven before leaving for work if you suspect, "I may have left the oven on."

However, thoughts can affect undesirable patterns of behavior that can make it difficult to go about daily tasks, especially if they become obsessive (recurring). Checking repeatedly can result from the obsessive thought, "I've left the oven on."

Obsessions or compulsions (acts done to ease the suffering or neutralize the idea), or both, are present in people with obsessive-compulsive disorder (OCD), an anxiety condition.

Some of the signs and symptoms of OCD include:

Cleanliness – obsessive handwashing or household cleaning to reduce an exaggerated fear of contamination; obsession with order or symmetry.

Safety Checking – obsessive fears about harm occurring to either themselves or others which can result in compulsive behaviors such as repeatedly checking whether the stove has been turned off or that windows and doors are locked.

Panic Disorder

When someone has a panic attack, they experience various physical symptoms as well as strong, overpowering, and frequently uncontrollable feelings of anxiety. Shortness of breath, chest pain, dizziness, and heavy sweating are all signs of a panic attack. People who are undergoing a panic attack may believe they are going to pass away or are having a heart attack. A person is said to have panic disorder if they experience recurring panic attacks or have a persistent worry of having one for longer than a month.

Post-Traumatic Stress Disorder (PTSD)

A specific set of reactions known as post-traumatic stress disorder (PTSD) can appear in persons who have experienced a traumatic event that put their lives, safety, or those around them in danger. It could be caused by a violent act or sexual assault, war or torture, or a natural disaster like a tornado, flood, or fire. The person feels terrible fear, helplessness, or horror.

Social Phobia

Social interactions and public speaking can cause severe anxiety for those with social phobia, referred to as social anxiety disorder. Even in everyday events, they fear being criticized, laughed at, or humiliated in front of others. For some persons with social phobia, dining in front of others at a restaurant might be terrifying.

DIFFERENCE BETWEEN ANXIETY AND ANXIETY DISORDER

Anxiety	Anxiety Disorder
Worrying about paying bills, landing a job, a romantic breakup, or other important life events.	Constant and unsubstantiated worry that causes significant distress and interferes with daily life.
Embarrassment or self-consciousness in an uncomfortable or awkward social situation.	Avoiding social situations for fear of being judged, embarrassed, or humiliated.
A case of nerves or sweating before a big business presentation, stage performance, or other significant events.	Seemingly out-of-the-blue panic attacks and preoccupation with the fear of having another.
Realistic fear of a dangerous object, place, or situation.	Irrational fear or avoidance of an object, place, or situation that poses little or no threat of danger.
Anxiety, sadness, or difficulty sleeping immediately after a traumatic event.	Recurring nightmares, flashbacks, or emotional numbing related to a traumatic event that occurred several months or years ago.

HABITS THAT MAKE ANXIETY WORSE

SKIPPING MEALS

Skipping meals causes hypoglycemia which can lead to symptoms such as irritability, nervousness, dizziness, light-headedness, and weakness.

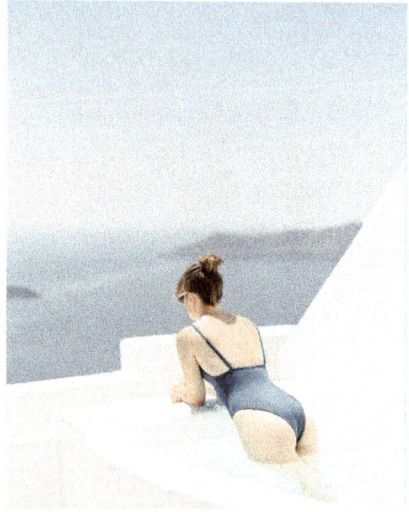

REACHING FOR SUGAR

Sugar has the ability to temporarily suppress anxiety and tension. Still, studies show that it increases the risk of anxiety and depression, and other health problems and diseases, which can worsen anxiety over time.

EATING POORLY

Poor eating habits can affect your intake of essential nutrients necessary for mental health and the functioning of the nervous system.

NOT EXERCISING

Your body is designed to move, and if you sit down all day and never exercise, your anxiety will likely increase.

WATCHING THE NEWS

Anxiety is characterized by excessive fear and worry, and watching the news can exacerbate that problem, leaving you feeling moody and anxious afterward.

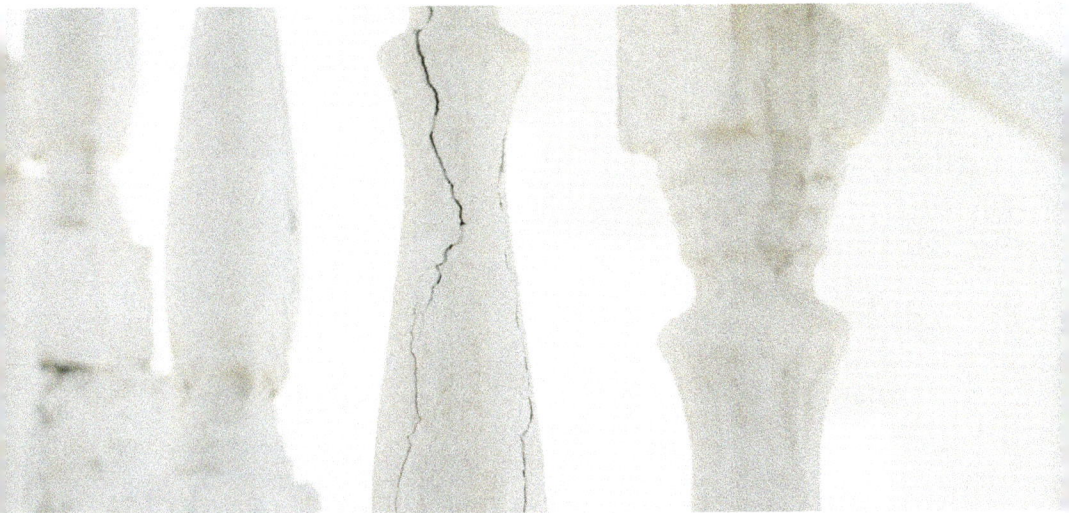

IGNORING YOUR ANXIETY

Anxiety is your body's way of indicating that something needs to change. Ignoring it will make anxiety worse.

DRINKING CAFFEINE

Caffeine is an "anxiety amplifier" that often affects anxiety hours later, making it difficult to realize the connection between the two.

EATING PROCESSED FOODS

According to research, processed foods contain additives that can increase anxiety while affecting a person's mood and social behavior.

NOT SLEEPING ENOUGH

Getting less than eight hours of sleep can increase repetitive negative thoughts and make it harder to let go of negative stuff—symptoms that are characteristics of anxiety.

"Various mechanisms can be used to deliver essential oils to target sites in the body. Typical routes of administration include inhalation, topical, and ingestion."

05 /

HEALTHY COPING MECHANISMS

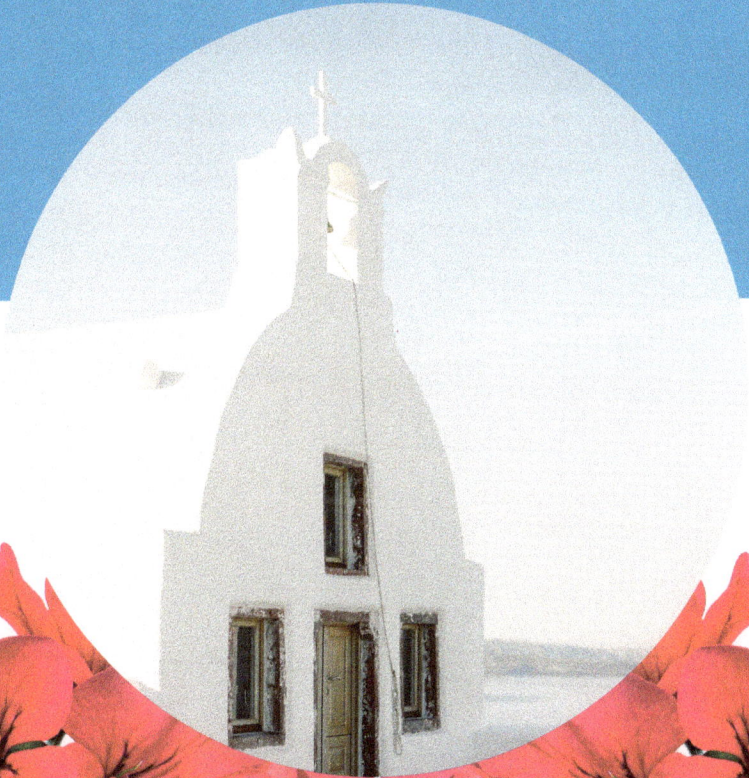

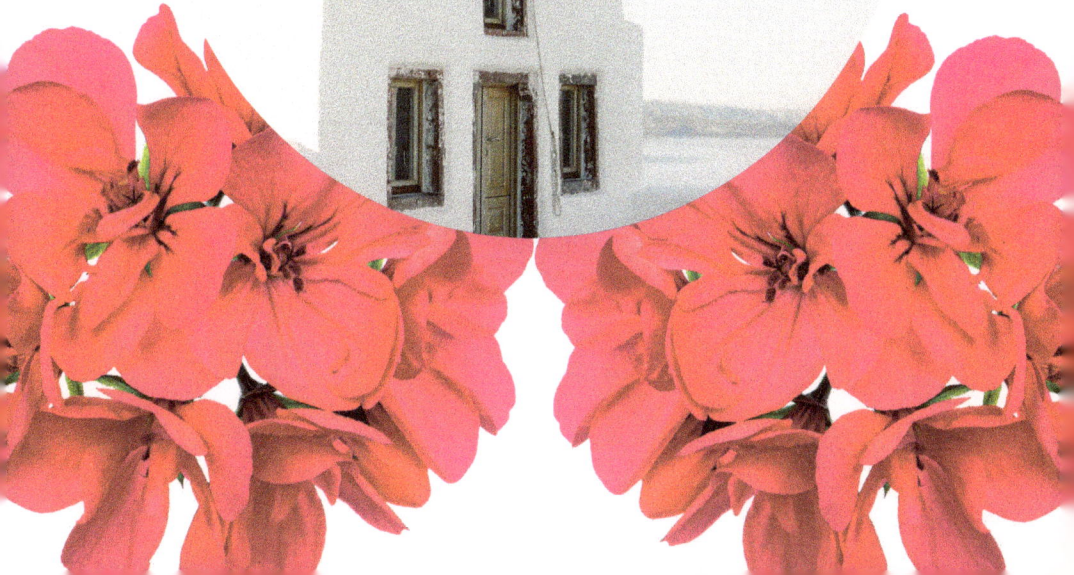

IDENTIFY WHAT IS BOTHERING YOU

You will need to identify what's upsetting you to address your anxiety's underlying cause. You will want to set aside time to examine your emotions and thoughts to accomplish this.

STOP AND BREATHE

Take a break whenever your anxiety attacks, and consider what is causing you to feel anxious. Typical anxiety symptoms include concern about a recent or future event.

The next time your nervousness starts to distract you from the moment, sit down and take a few deep breaths of an essential oil to reclaim your concentration. You can regain your sense of equilibrium and return to yourself by pausing for a moment and breathing.

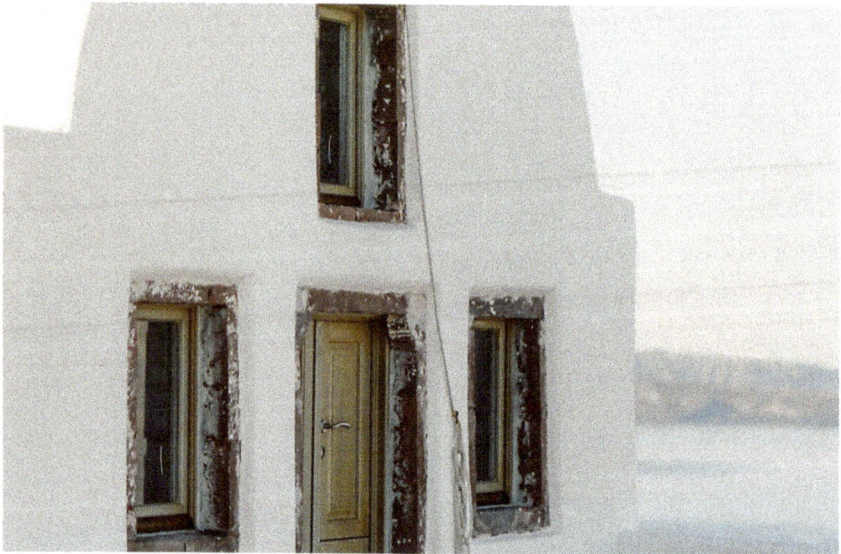

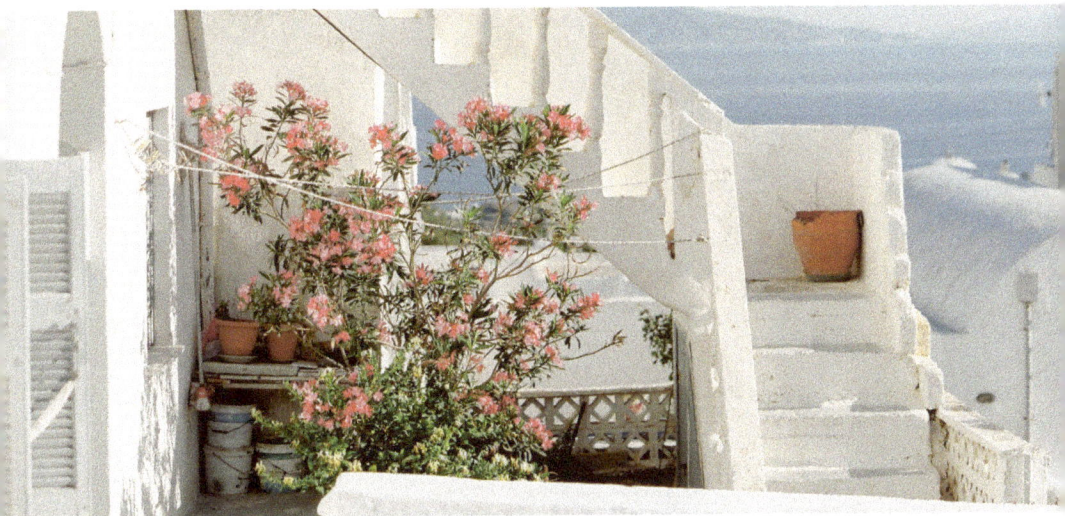

UNDERSTAND THINGS YOU CAN CHANGE

Anxiety is often caused by worrying about events that haven't even happened. Even if everything is fine, you could worry about future problems like losing your job, being sick, or ensuring the safety of your loved ones.

No matter how hard you try, life can be unpredictable, and you can't always control what happens. You can, however, choose how you will approach the unknowable. By letting go of fear and putting your attention on thankfulness, you can use your worry as a power source.

Anxiety is often caused by worrying about events that haven't even happened.

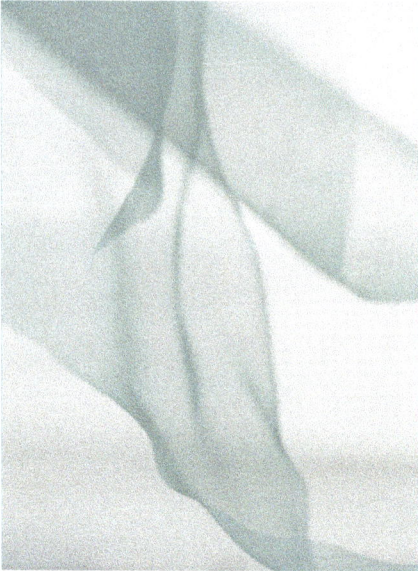

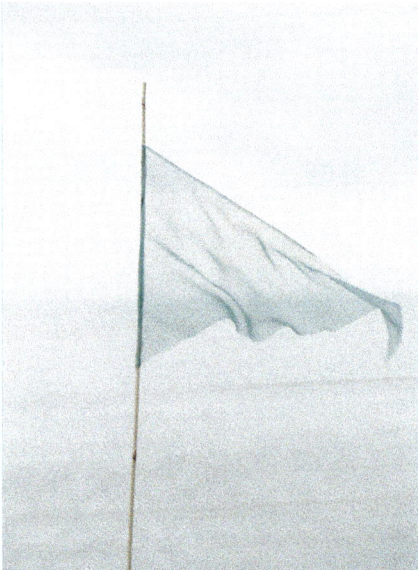

STRENGTHEN YOUR MIND AND BRAIN

Changes in your way of life can also be beneficial for preventing anxiety and assisting you in coping with anxiety attacks. Your degree of physical activity, how much sleep you get, and what you eat can all affect how anxious you feel.

According to research, your mood and stress levels can be impacted by what you eat. For instance, those who consume diets high in fruits and vegetables tend to have lower stress levels.

Your mental health and anxiety levels can both be significantly impacted by sleep. According to research, sleep issues, particularly with those who suffer from generalized anxiety disorder, have been linked to an increased risk of stress and anxiety. Even brief, poor sleep can have this effect.

MASTER YOUR ANXIETY

- Instead of letting anxiety take over, note it as soon as you feel it.
- Once you recognize it, you can explore its source.
- Try writing down your worries, getting as granular to the root cause as possible.
- Narrow down your thoughts and anxious feelings to set realistic concerns.
- Create a plan of action to manage anxiety, solve problems, and accept things you can't change.
- Sit with your emotions and allow any feelings to exist alongside whatever actionable steps you're taking.
- Once you take appropriate action and know what you're doing, it'll help you calm down.

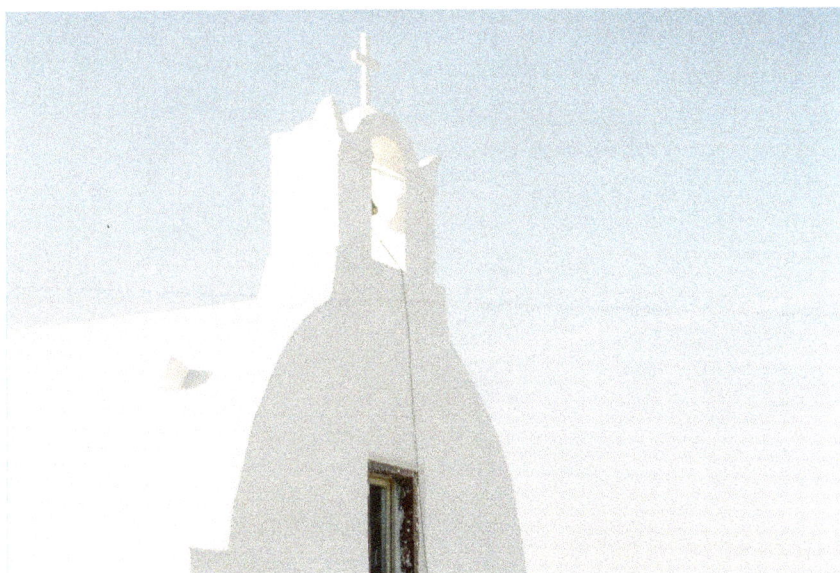

HOW TO DEAL WITH ANXIETY

Get Professional Help

If you struggle with anxiety or depression, involving a medical or mental health professional can be helpful. This can be an important step if you struggle to make any changes in your life to begin addressing the symptoms that you're experiencing.

Practice Deep Breathing

While there are several different types of deep breathing techniques, you don't need a specific strategy to benefit from this. You can focus on taking slow, deep breaths through your nose, holding it for a few seconds, and then slowly breathing out through your mouth.

Develop a Sleep Schedule

Working to get on a sleep schedule may help address this problem. Most adults should get between seven and nine hours of sleep a night. Focus on trying to sleep at the same time each night and waking up at the same time each morning. This can help your body adjust to the new routine.

Focus on taking slow, deep breaths through your nose, then slowly breathing out through your mouth.

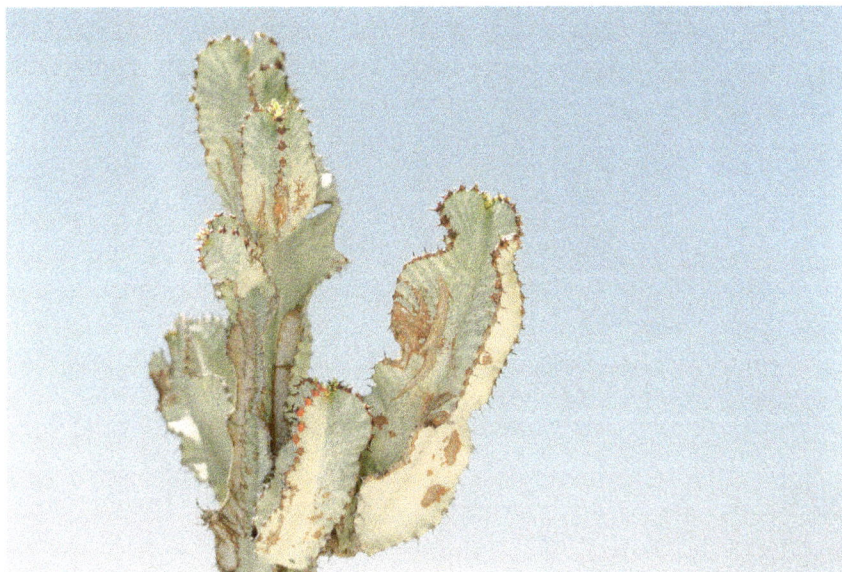

Set Simple Goals for the Day

Depending on the impact of anxiety on you, these goals can be straightforward, such as making your bed when you wake up or eating lunch at a particular time of the day. Doing this can help set you up for success, and when you start to have these small victories, it can help you feel more energized to tackle slightly larger tasks.

Pay Attention to What You're Eating

The food you eat can have a significant impact on the way you feel and your energy levels. Many people turn to caffeine or sugary drinks and snacks if they feel their energy dip. However, this can have the opposite impact on your psyche.

Turn to Your Support System

It can be helpful to build a strong support system around yourself. This could be made up of family and friends, or you could join a support group of others going through similar experiences. This can be helpful to have people that care about you who can check in on you to see how you're doing.

Exercise

Engaging in physical activity can release chemicals in your brain that help boost your mood. It also helps prepare your body for taking action. The good news is you don't have to be engaged in a rigorous exercise regimen to benefit from this.

Go Outside

You may not have the energy to tackle your to-do list for the day or jump into a workout, but even going outside can help improve your energy levels. You may even notice less stress and lower blood pressure when you spend more time outdoors.

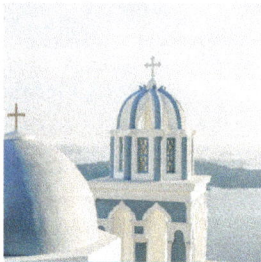

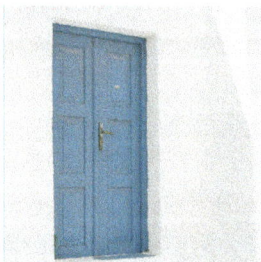

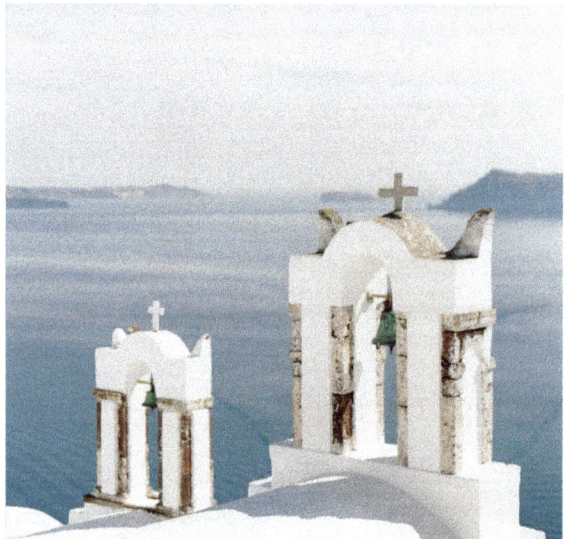

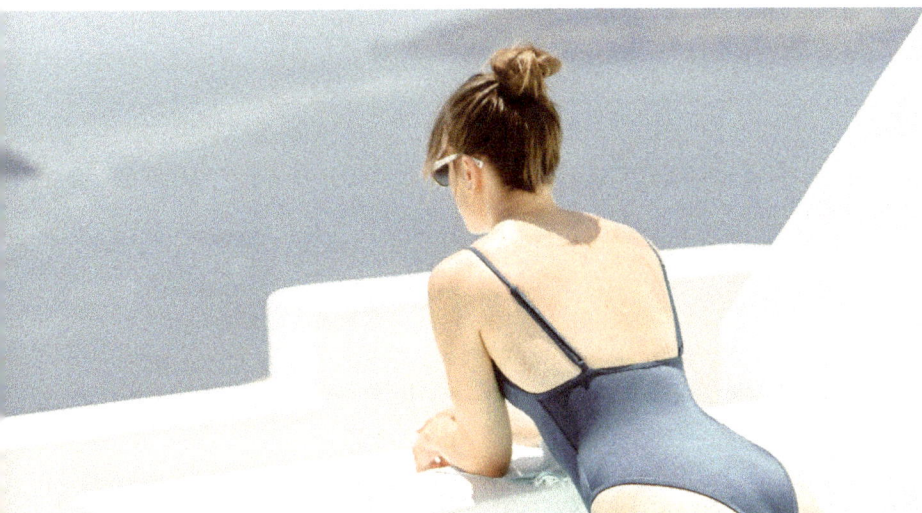

Journaling

You may experience an increase in energy levels through journaling. Writing down your thoughts and concerns in a journal can help you relieve some of the anxious thoughts running through your mind.

If you keep a journal, you can track your anxiety symptoms. You can tell the doctor or counselor, "I suffer from anxiety, and these are my symptoms." Once this first step has been made, it can give you a sense of achievement that you are beginning to take back control of your life and feelings. It will be a journey to recovery, but you have taken the first step.

So now it is time to plan for the next step of your journey by identifying your triggers and making a plan on how to deal with those triggers.

Journaling about your symptoms can give you a sense of achievement that you are beginning to take back control of your life and feelings.

Physical Activity

Research shows that physical activity such as regular walking—not just formal exercise programs—may help improve mood. Physical activity and exercise are not the same, but both benefit your health.

Physical activity works your muscles and requires energy, including work, household, or leisure activities. At the same time, exercise is a planned, structured, repetitive body movement to improve or maintain physical fitness.

The word "exercise" may make you think of running laps around the gym. But exercise includes many activities that boost your activity level to help you feel better.

Indeed, running, lifting weights, playing basketball, and other fitness activities that get your heart pumping can help. But so can physical activity such as gardening, washing your car, walking around the block, or engaging in other less intense activities. Any physical activity that gets you off the couch and moving can help improve your mood.

You don't have to do all your exercise or other physical activity at once. Broaden how you think of exercise and find ways to add small amounts of physical activity throughout your day. For example, take the stairs instead of the elevator. Park a little farther away from work to fit in a short walk. Or, if you live close to your job, consider biking to work.

Find ways to add small amounts of physical activity throughout the day.

LIFESTYLE CHANGES FOR REDUCING ANXIETY

Adopt Healthy Eating Habits

Adopting healthy eating habits helps reduce anxiety, lift mood, and improve overall physical health.

Give Importance to Sleep

While sleeping, your body supports healthy brain function and maintains physical and mental health.

Exercise Daily

Taking part in daily physical activity is another lifestyle change that can transform your life and anxiety levels.

Meditation Routine

Meditating in the morning is very important to relieve your anxiety and start your day feeling calm.

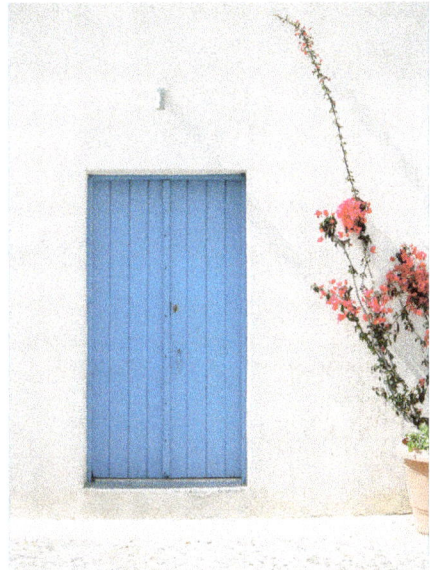

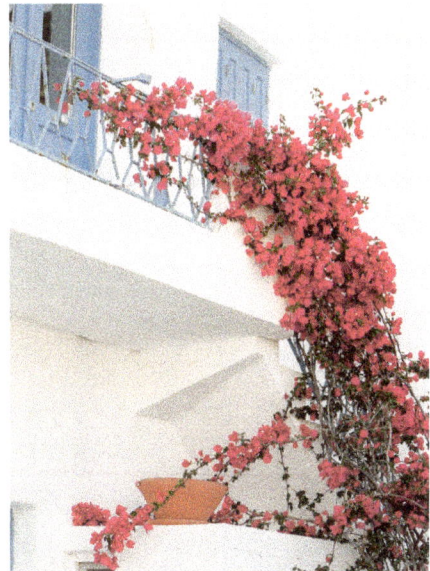

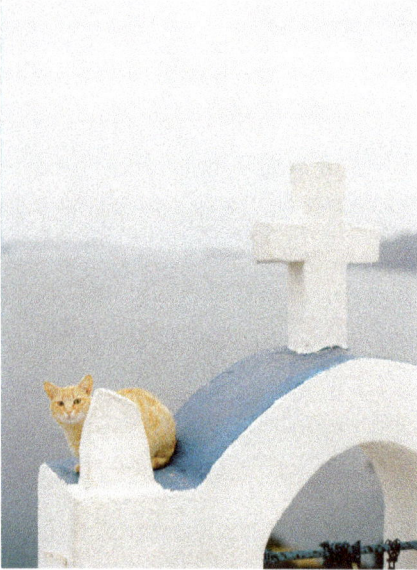

Regularly Express Emotions

Finding a way to express your emotions regularly can help you reduce your anxiety.

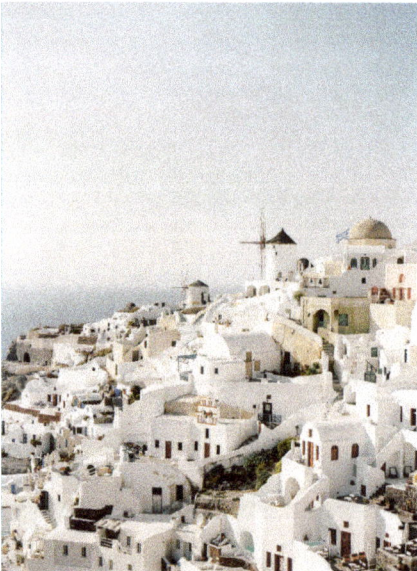

Simplify Your Life

Dealing with anxiety is challenging and overwhelming. But often, we make our life more complicated than it needs to be, which makes anxiety worse.

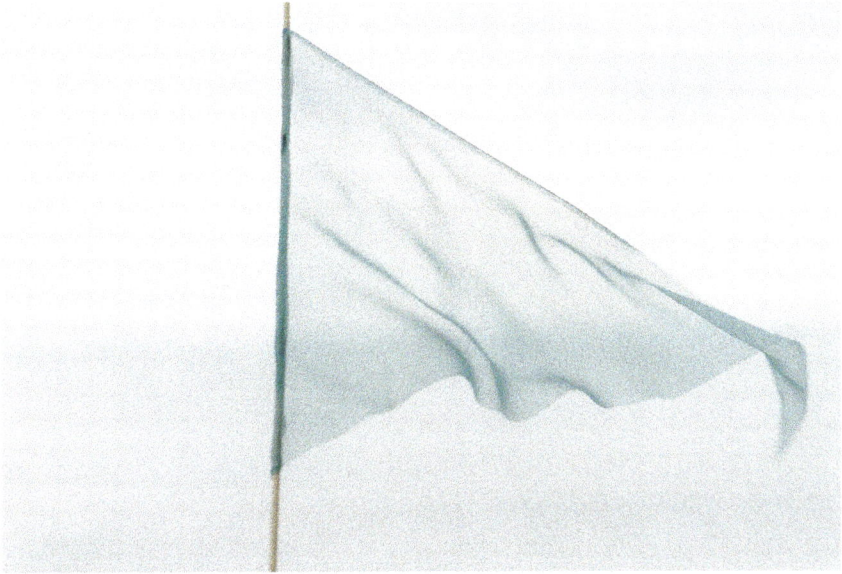

Therapeutic Movements

Any activity that involves purposeful movements can be thera-peutic. It isn't like your everyday movements while making tea or loading the dishwasher.

Therapeutic movements are done on purpose while you are fully aware of your body and how it is feeling. During this activity, your mind is focused on your body, muscles, and bones.

Any purposeful movement that you can comfortably do can be therapeutic. For example, you could stretch your arms upwards and feel the muscle stretching in your arms and shoulders.

Try setting aside fifteen minutes every day to do some therapeu-tic movements where you focus on your body. Bending, stretch-ing, and twisting are good movements as long as they don't hurt. You could also watch some simple yoga instructional videos on YouTube.

Unhelpful Thoughts

When a person experiences an unhelpful emotion, such as depression or anxiety, it is usually preceded by several unhelpful self-statements and thoughts.

Unhelpful emotions, such as depression or anxiety, are usually preceded by several unhelpful self-statements or thoughts.

Catastrophizing – Exaggerating a situation in the negative.

All or Nothing – Absolute thinking focusing on extremes. There is no in-between.

Emotional Reasoning – Interpreting current emotions as fact.

Mental Filter – Focusing on only one aspect of a situation (often negative) while overlooking others (positive).

Magnification and Minimization – Magnifying the positives in others while minimizing your own.

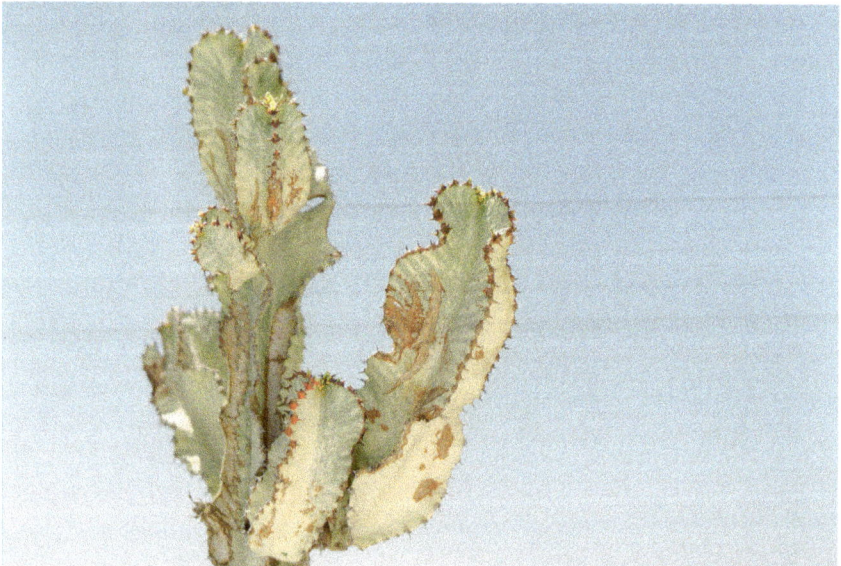

Unhelpful Thinking Styles

Jumping to Conclusions – Not waiting for an explanation.

Mind Reading – Assuming we know someone else's thoughts or motives.

Predictive Thinking – Overestimating negative emotions or outcomes.

Labeling – Using sweeping, negative statements to describe yourself or others.

Personalization – Blaming yourself unnecessarily for external negative events.

Overgeneralizing – Interpreting a single, negative event as the norm or enduring pattern.

Should-have and Must-have Statements – Putting unreasonable expectations on oneself.

Once you take the first step, you will be on the journey to recovery.

OTHER HELPFUL THOUGHT TIPS

1. Stopping and interrupting a thought as it begins. Use a strong image or a word to interrupt the thought. Firmly state it, either internally or aloud.

2. Distracting. Redirect your mind to something else internally or externally, preferably something pleasant and engaging.

3. Mindful observing. Watch, label, or log your thoughts. Use the language "I am thinking..." or "My mind is having the thought that..." to distance yourself from the thought.

4. Understanding. Begin to understand where thoughts come from by asking several questions, including "What is the purpose of this thought?" and "Does it tie to a specific schema?"

5. Mindfully letting go. Use imagery or words to visualize thoughts passing by. Good examples are clouds in the sky or leaves on a stream.

6. Having gratitude. Focus on something you are grateful for from the past, present, or future.

HOW OVERCOMING ANXIETY WILL CHANGE YOUR LIFE

Unraveling anxiety might feel like you're exposing yourself to more pain. However, the outcome is worth it. Below is a list of ways that overcoming anxiety will change your life.

- Your life goals will be easier to achieve. When you are no longer fearful and avoiding situations, you will feel free to pursue that promotion or take that once-in-a-lifetime trip. Goals that seemed out of reach will suddenly become realistic.

- You will think more positively about your future. Anxiety tends to cast a negative outlook on what is yet to come. When you are free of anxiety, you will feel more hopeful about what is around the next corner.

- It will be easier to cope with medical conditions. You won't worry unnecessarily about your physical health but will do what is necessary to take care of yourself. Visits to the doctor will no longer fill you with anxiety and dread.

- You may feel relief from depression or low mood. When anxiety is relieved, depression and low mood often show improvement as well. Along with feeling less anxious, you may feel more optimistic, have more energy, sleep better, and generally have more interest in life.

- Anxiety will no longer define you as a person. If you have long-held beliefs about yourself that center around being anxious, those will be replaced with feelings of self-esteem and self-worth. You will get to know the person you can be without those anxious thoughts.

- You will take better care of yourself. Overcoming anxiety will shed light on areas of your life that have been neglected. You will give more importance to nutrition, exercise, and being present in the moment.

- Relationships and work that have suffered will improve. You might develop new social connections or feel less dependent on people you have previously leaned on. Your increased ability to concentrate will make work seem like less of a chore, and you might even find yourself seeking advancement in the workplace.

- You will feel increased enjoyment in life and more confidence. Anxiety has a way of zapping your confidence and happiness. If you've felt like every day you were just "getting through," you will now start each day confidently.

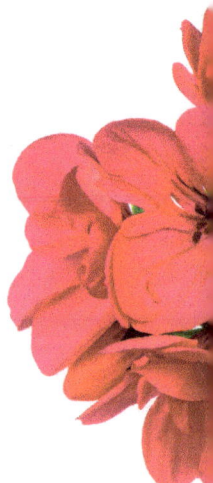

ROUTINES AND COMFORT

An excellent way to prevent anxiety from taking hold is to have a healthy routine. Knowing what you are doing for some of your day is comforting. This section looks at how you can make a routine for yourself.

Having a healthy routine does not mean you must be regimented and have all your activities timed and done to the letter. No! It means organizing part of your day in a way that is comfortable for you. You design your routine for your comfort and not anyone else's. It also means that you know what will happen during parts of your day, and that small amount of predictability brings peace of mind.

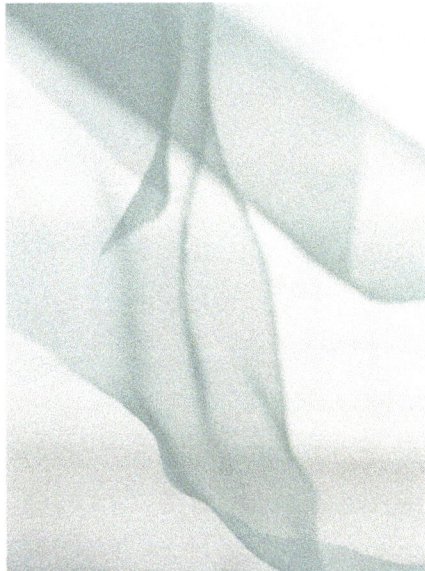

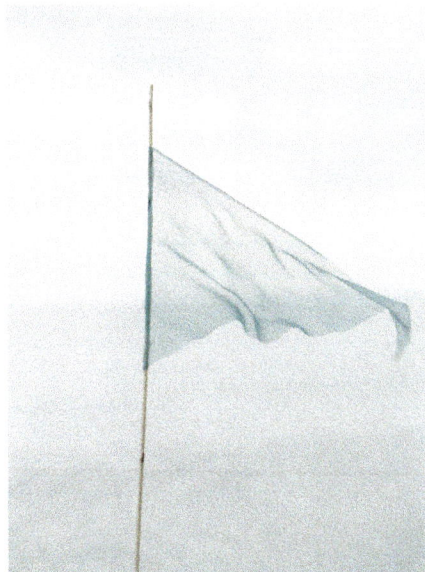

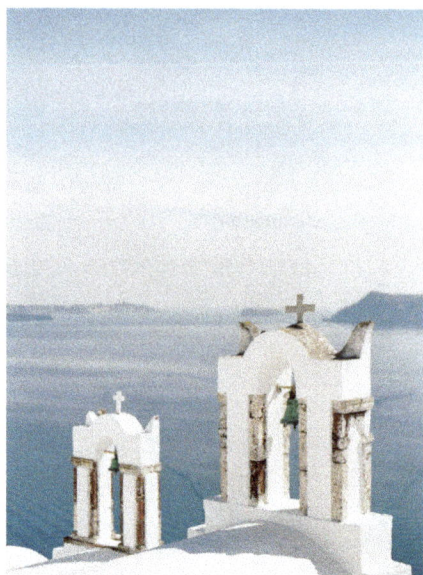

For example: When you first wake up, you need time to gather your thoughts and set the tone for the day. Try setting your alarm fifteen minutes before you usually get up so that you can have five minutes of thinking before going and getting yourself a drink. While having your drink, think about positive things, such as three things you are grateful for or three things that you like about yourself.

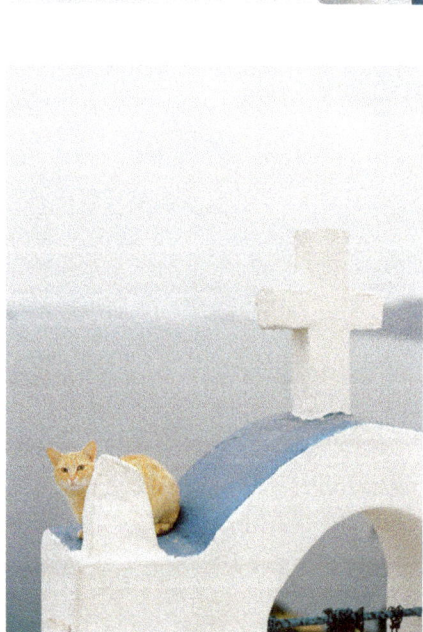

Don't start your day by thinking about everything you have to do or any worries you have. Doing that will set you up for tension and negativity.

Plan your day to have at least times when you can have some "you" time. This might be during lunch or after you finish work in a hot bath.

Do not fill up your day doing things for work or other people. You deserve time to yourself.

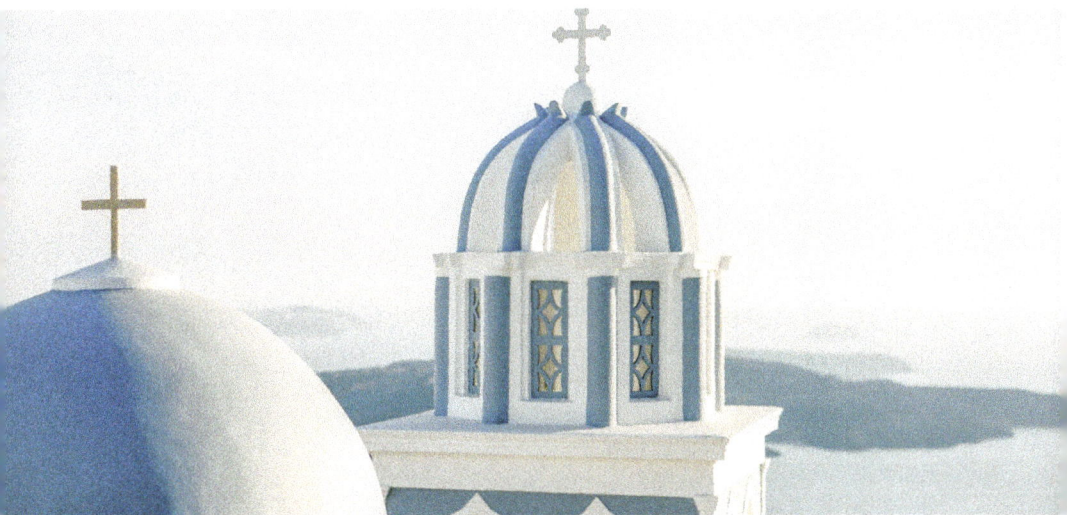

1. 15-Minute Meditation

Try a simple meditation for 15 minutes or more. Search YouTube for short, powerful meditations.

2. Deep Breathing

This is simple, but it works. Breathe deeply for four counts, hold your breath for four counts, and exhale for four counts. Do this until you feel clear-minded and less emotional.

3. Talk It Out Mentally

Make a list of three or more people to whom you can express your anxious feelings.

If you suddenly and unexpectedly feel joy, don't hesitate. Give in to it. — Mary Oliver

4. Write!

Take a notebook out and write down your worries until you feel satisfied. Which concerns are you going to let go of today?

5. A Tech Detox

Don't touch your phone, laptop, or iPad for one hour or more. You can spend this time reading, taking a bath, exercising, or creating something.

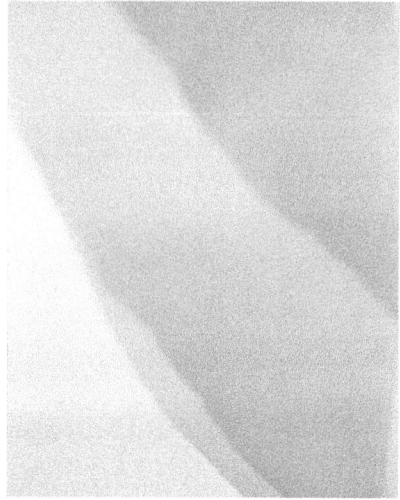

6. Get Moving

If you are having anxious thoughts, get up and do a household chore, do some yoga, bake, go walking, or do anything which moves your body.

7. Plan and Prepare

Planning is the best way to prevent anxious feelings. Plan your time, and prepare for your day the night before. Start the day knowing exactly what you need to accomplish!

8. Mindful Activities

Choose an activity that lets you be present in the moment for at least one hour, such as painting, writing, reading, window shopping, or drinking coffee at a cafe. Don't multitask!

DECLUTTER THE MIND

WHAT IS DECLUTTERING?

The dictionary definition of decluttering is the removal of unnecessary items from an untidy or overcrowded space.

The process can be applied to tangible physical items in your home or workplace, such as books, furniture, and clothes.

Decluttering can also be applied to intangible things that constantly occupy your mind, such as negative thoughts, worries, and responsibilities. A calendar crammed with too many commitments, or people making unnecessary demands on your time and attention, can become overwhelming and cause anxiety.

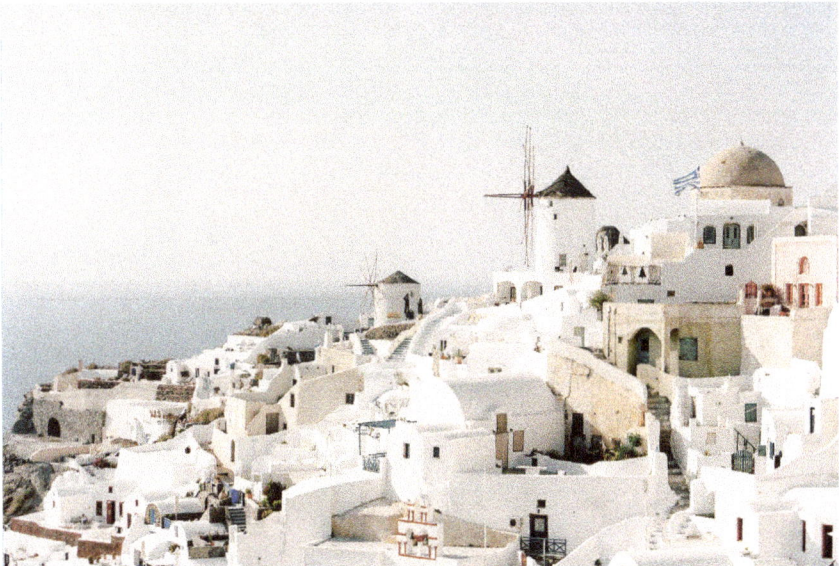

Understanding Decluttering of the Mind

There's something worse than having a cluttered home or work space, and that's having a cluttered mind. A cluttered mind is restless and unfocused. It tries to move in many different directions at once, and the result is that very little gets done.

Many of us suffer from having too much on our minds! You might be worried about the future, reflecting on past regrets, or fretting about a long mental to-do list. When your mind is so busy with different thoughts, it isn't easy to focus and be productive.

Everything can seem overwhelming, and it often leads to feelings of anxiety or panic.

You might be suffering from disturbed sleep as a result, which in turn exacerbates the problem as you become more tired. (For more on this, read my book, *Sleep Well With Essential Oil,* to learn more about the importance of sleep.)

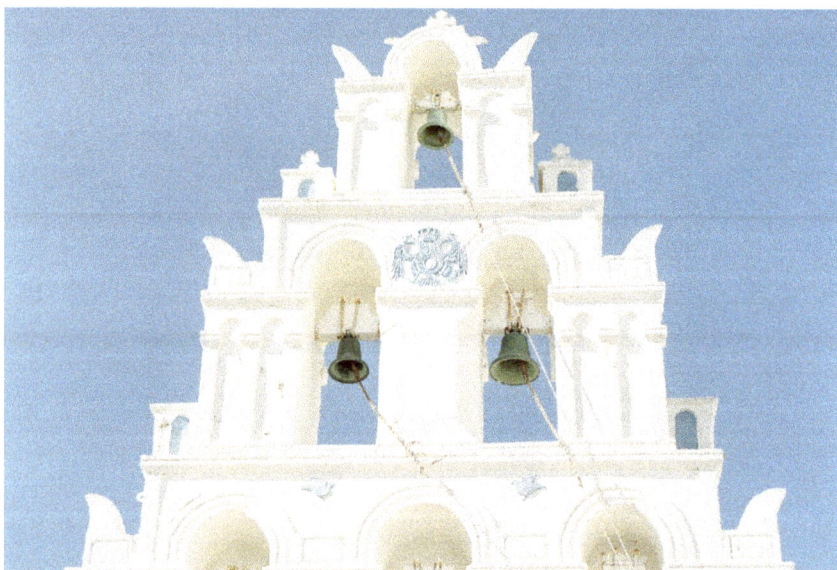

Mental clutter can include worrying about the future, ruminating about the past, keeping a mental to-do list, complaints, etc. Fortunately, you can use strategies and techniques to clean out some space in your head.

DECLUTTERING THE MIND TECHNIQUES

Declutter Your Home or Workspace

A cluttered home or work-space leads to a cluttered mind. Cluttered surround-ings constantly tell your brain that there is stuff to be done; organizing, cleaning, tidying. The brain feels bombarded by the stimulus, causing stress and anxiety.

Write Things Down

Keep your journal or notepad nearby so that if your con-centration is interrupted by a sudden thought you need to remember, you can write it down for later and carry on with what you were doing.

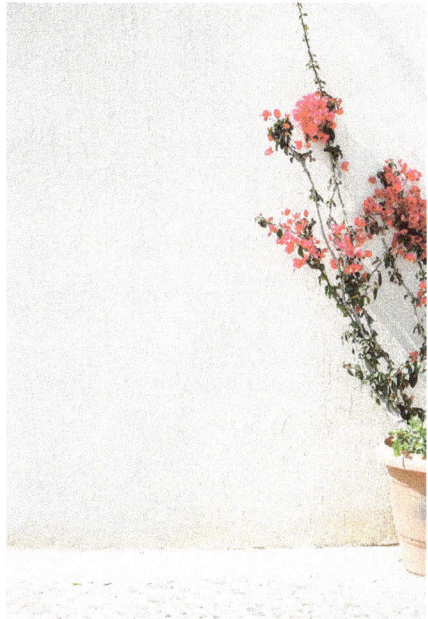

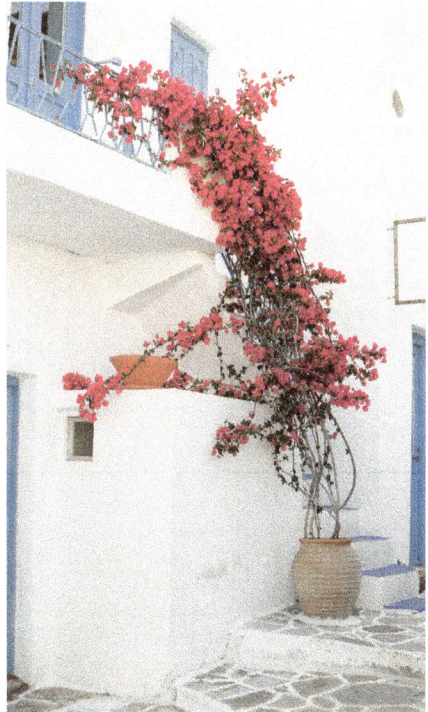

Stop Multitasking and Prioritize

Set aside a specific amount of time in which you can focus entirely on one particular important task. Keep all other mental clutter out of your headspace while you are concentrating on the task at hand. Break down your larger mental clutter into smaller chunks that are easier to tackle individually.

Be Decisive and Don't Feel Awkward About Saying No

Don't feel under obligation to attend social events because you think you should. Choose engagements that are worth your time and energy. Spend time with the people who boost your mental well-being.

Don't Dwell on the Past and Don't Worry About What You Can Control

Worrying is a waste of valuable mental energy. Worrying doesn't make anything better. It clutters your mind and makes you feel worse. You have control over the problem and then do the things you can to change it. If you can, then let it go.

Anxiety is a thin stream of fear trickling through the mind. If encouraged, it cuts a channel to which all other thoughts are drained.

06 / WHAT IS AN ESSENTIAL OIL?

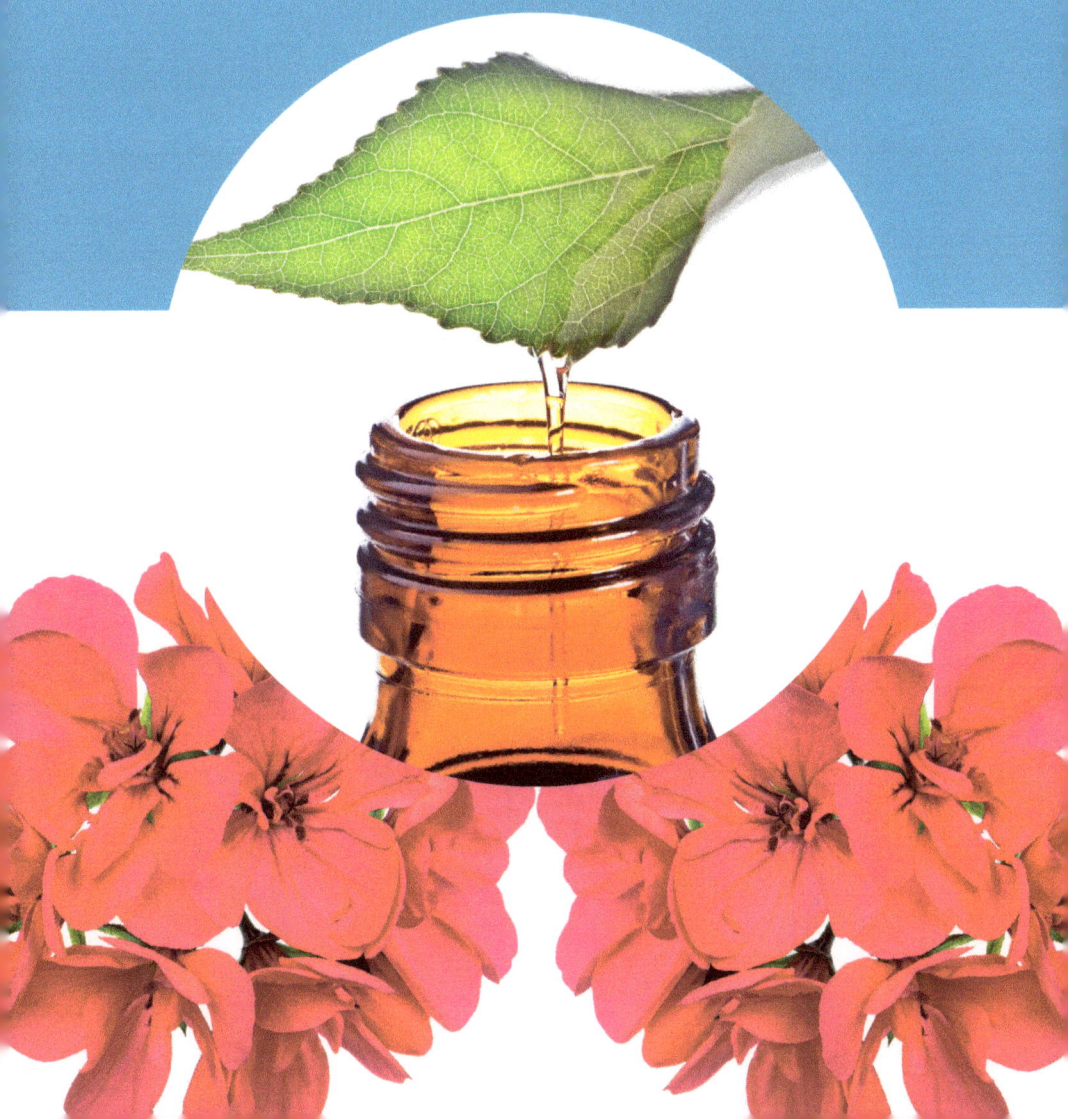

Essential oils are fragrant, vital fluids distilled from flowers, shrubs, leaves, trees, roots, and seeds. Because they are necessary for the life of the plant and play a vital role in the biological processes of the vegetation, these substances are called "essential." They carry the lifeblood, intelligence, and vibrational energy that endow them with the healing power to sustain their own life—and help the people who use them.

All essential oils have unique medicinal properties, characteristics, and therapeutic benefits that will differ depending on the soil, climate, and altitude of the countries where the plants were grown.

Today, oils are used in aromatherapy to promote well-being and good health. While the term aromatherapy can seem ambiguous, "scent" is only one aspect of aromatherapy, as you will discover many more dramatic benefits for healing the body, mind, and spirit.

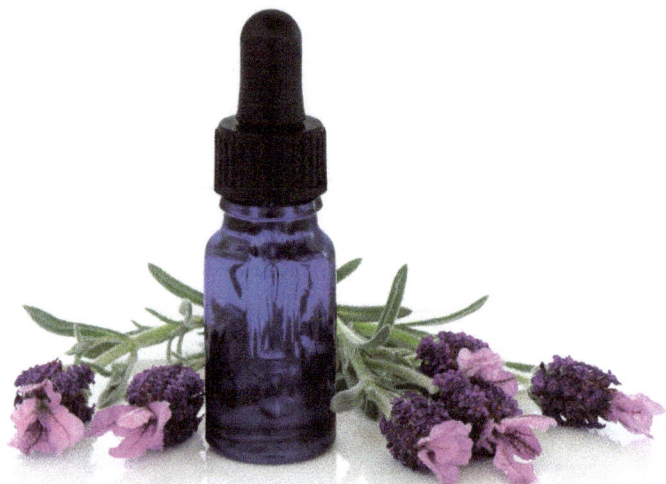

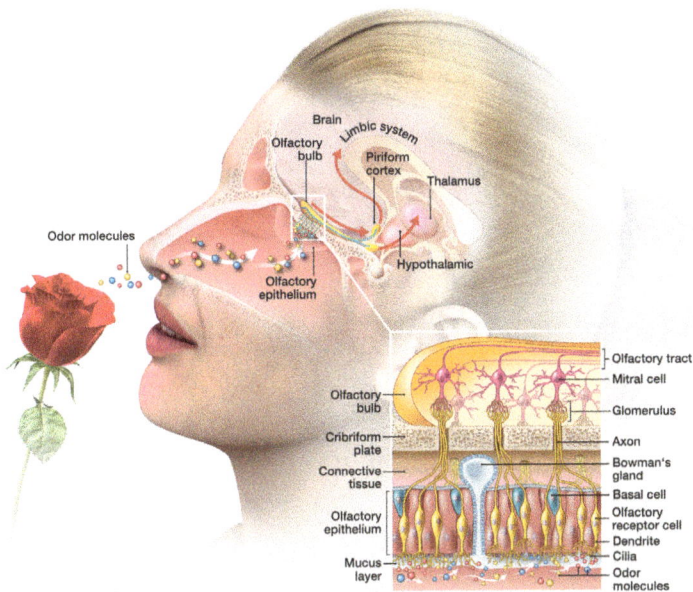

Figure labels: Brain, Limbic system, Olfactory bulb, Piriform cortex, Thalamus, Hypothalamic, Odor molecules, Olfactory epithelium

Inset labels: Olfactory tract, Mitral cell, Olfactory bulb, Glomerulus, Cribriform plate, Axon, Connective tissue, Bowman's gland, Basal cell, Olfactory epithelium, Olfactory receptor cell, Dendrite, Cilia, Mucus layer, Odor molecules

HOW ESSENTIAL OILS WORK

When essential oils are diffused in the air, the nose, wired differently than the other four senses, carries the oil's molecules directly into the head via the olfactory system. The olfactory membranes, with almost 800 million nerve endings, receive the micro-fine, vaporized oil particles and carry them along the axon of the nerve fibers, connecting them with the secondary neurons in the olfactory bulb. The sense of smell facilitated through the olfactory nerve invites the fragrance of essential oils into some areas of the brain, which enables the body to process them naturally. The scent molecules stimulate the brain's limbic region, pineal gland, and pituitary gland. Of the five human senses, the sense of smell is the only one that is directly connected to the brain.

The olfactory system, closely linked to the limbic system, dramatically influences the body's physiology. Research has shown that these aromatic compounds can exert strong effects on the brain, especially on the hypothalamus (the hormone command center of the body) and the limbic system (the seat of emotions). Molecules that pass through the blood-brain barrier and

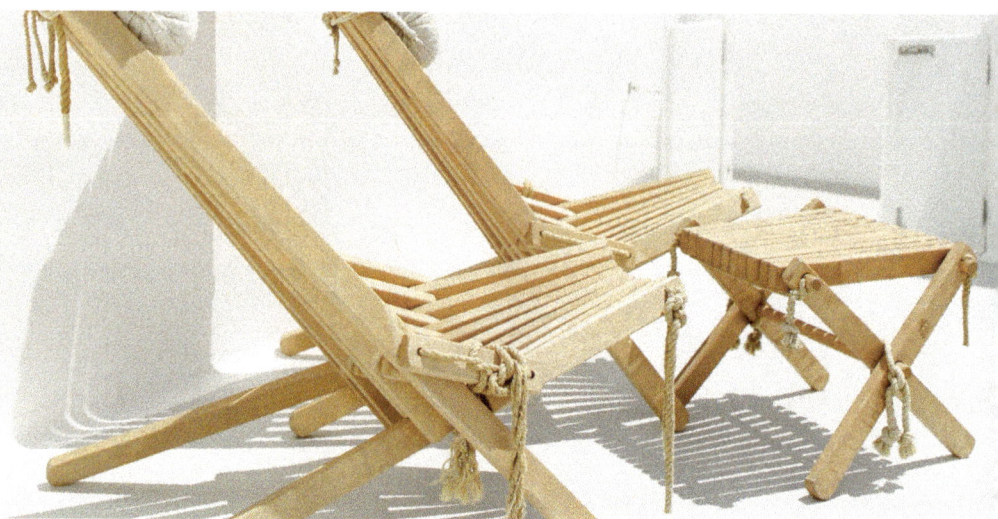

stimulate various constituents of the brain can exert their effect quickly and result in stress relief and sleep promotion. This knowledge has been used to treat multiple conditions, such as anxiety, and to provide relief for chronic pain.

The limbic system, which is directly linked to those areas of the brain that control our memory, blood pressure, heart rate, hormone balance, breathing, and stress levels, can be significantly influenced by essential oils, which can reach the limbic system by bypassing the cerebral cortex. This is important in that once inhaled, they affect the physiological and psychological function of the body with positive results. Therapeutic properties beneficial for the limbic system include antidepressant, calming, grounding, relaxing, and sedative.

Essential oils can significantly influence the physiological and psychological function of the body with positive results.

YOUR BRAIN ON ESSENTIAL OILS

People who experience stress daily may find using essential oils helpful for calming their nerves and promoting a less stressful environment. One of the reasons why aromatherapy works so well in this situation is that essential oils' molecules are easily inhaled, which allows them to be fast-acting and quickly absorbed into the body. The molecules released through aromatherapy stimulate and affect portions of the brain that can trigger specific emotions or soothe other less desirable emotions.

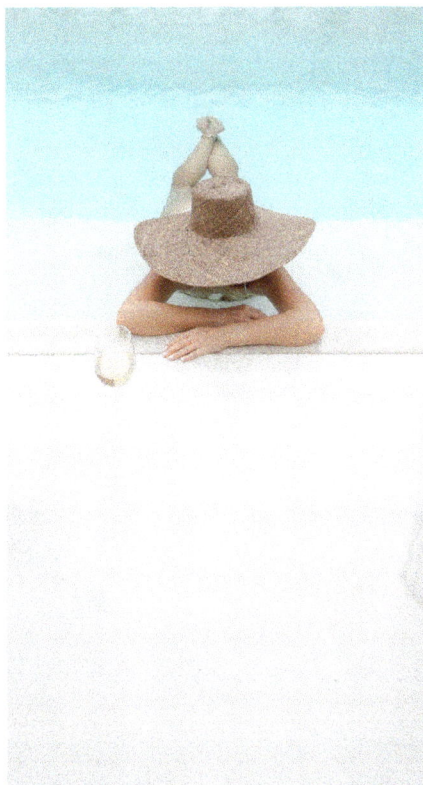

When essential oils are inhaled, molecules from the essential oils make their way to the brain, where they affect the amygdala, a part of the limbic system, also known as the emotional center of the brain.

Essential oils work through the olfactory system to cause the brain to secrete neurotransmitters, such as dopamine and serotonin, which can elevate one's mood. These neurotransmitters are necessary to make you feel calm and relaxed. Serotonin is also needed to produce melatonin, the hormone responsible for making you feel sleepy at bedtime.

When an essential oil contains any of the chemical properties listed above with a soothing, calming, or relaxing nature, it induces a positive response within the brain and the body. After inhaling an essential oil with calming properties, the brain processes the aroma, and a physical effect follows afterward.

The brain then positively associates that aroma, remembering it the next time it is used. The brain makes a connection with this aroma and, from then on, recognizes it. This particular oil with calming properties for anxiety can continue to be used because of this connection between it and the brain.

YOUR BODY ON ESSENTIAL OILS

Many studies have been conducted on aromatherapy's benefits in using essential oils to lessen anxiety. Research indicates that aromatherapy can modify anxiety symptoms in the brain's waves and behavior. Essential oils can block the neural connections that cause the body to release adrenaline and cortisol without need. For this reason, aromatherapy has become popular in reducing the perception of anxiousness by increasing contentment and decreasing cortisol levels, the "stress hormone."

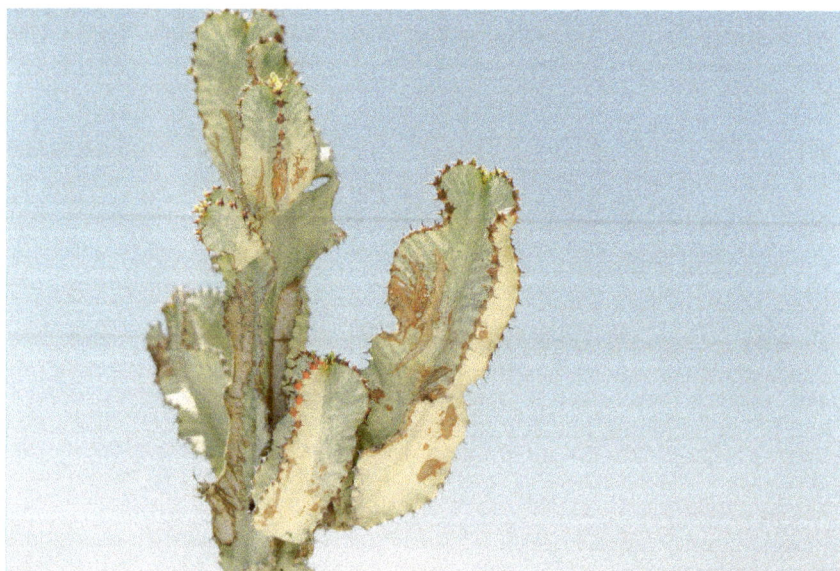

Certain essential oils trigger the release of certain neurochemicals and hormones, including serotonin which slows the heart rate, regulates blood pressure, and boosts the immune system, thereby reversing the effects of stress. While you may not always be able to prevent a negative situation, aromatherapy is an effective way to ease the emotional distress that accompanies stressful events. Reducing negative emotions can change how you think and act, reducing anxiousness.

For example, among the many benefits of Lavender essential oil is its ability to help a person relax due to its chemical molecule, linalool, which modulates the neurohormone GABA (gamma-aminobutyric acid). This, in turn, regulates adrenaline, noradrenaline, and dopamine levels.

The term "adaptogen" describes oils that can relax and stimulate as needed. By calming or stimulating body systems, they bring about homeostasis. Adaptogens help the body adapt to stress by restoring the adrenal glands, which can become overstimulated or exhausted by anxiety. Various essential oils are adaptogens, including Lavender, Rose, and Geranium.

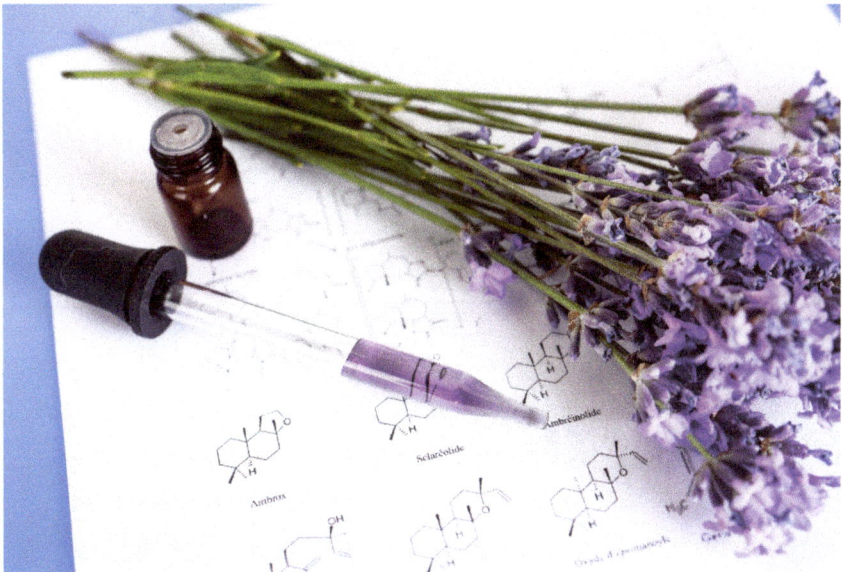

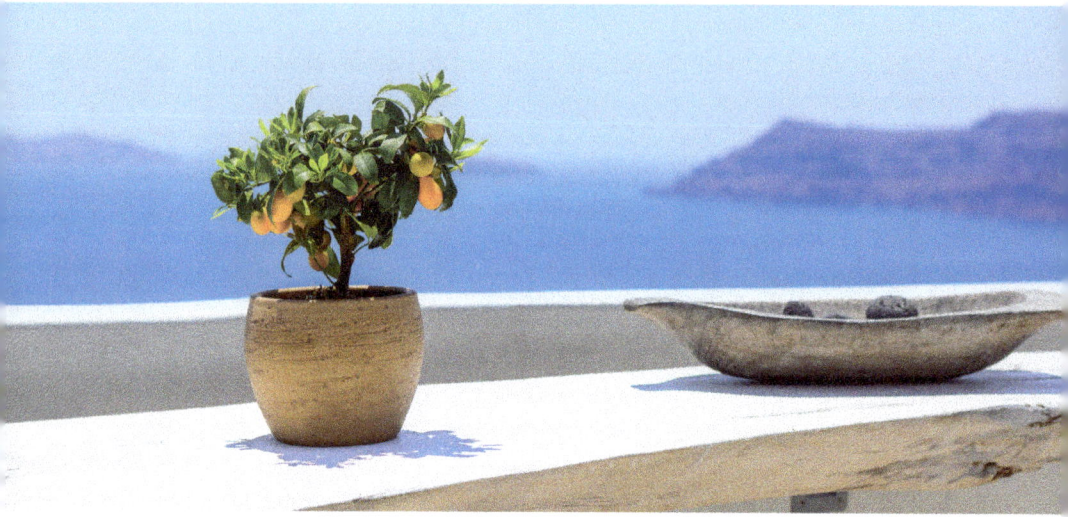

Essential oils are indispensable in helping people cope with anxiety and other emotional barriers. As mentioned earlier, linalool in Lavender reduces anxiety, while limonene, found in many citrus oils, can ease anxiety and depression. Chamomile and Bergamot essential oils contain the compounds alpha- and beta-pinene, which also work as antidepressants, helping to lift spirits and increase feelings of well-being.

Chemical constituents such as aldehydes and esters in certain essential oils can have a calming and soothing effect on the central nervous system (including both the sympathetic and parasympathetic systems). The hypothalamus and pituitary gland are then stimulated to produce neurochemicals, including serotonin plus the hormones that balance and regulate various body systems, such as the endocrine, immune, and nervous system. Because essential oils affect the amygdala and pineal gland in the brain, they

Chemical constituents such as aldehydes and esters in certain essential oils can have a calming and soothing effect on the central nervous system.

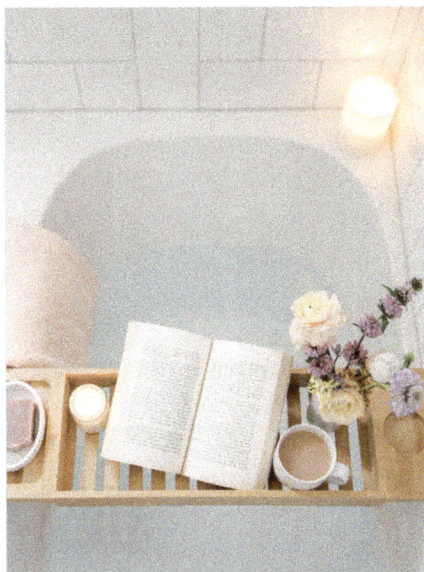

can help the mind and body release emotional trauma and sharpen focus.

Essential oils like Lavender and Chamomile allow us to relax instead of letting anxiety build up in our bodies, causing havoc. Unchecked anxiety creates an acidic condition that activates the transcript enzyme, transcribes that anxiety on the RNA template, and stores it in the DNA. That emotion then becomes a predominant factor in our lives from that moment on.

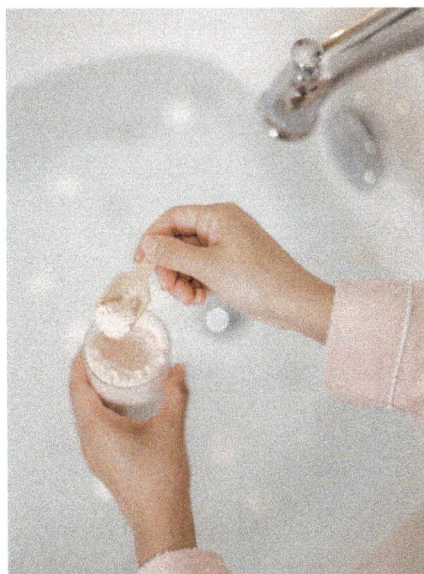

When we encounter an emotionally charged situation, instead of being overwhelmed by it, we can diffuse essential oils, put them in our bath, or wear them as cologne. The aromatic molecules will be absorbed into the bloodstream from the nasal cavity to the limbic system. The molecules activate the amygdala (the memory center for fear and trauma) and sedate and relax the sympathetic/parasympathetic system. The fragrant molecules help the body minimize the acid created so that it does not initiate a reaction with the transcript enzyme.

HOW ESSENTIAL OILS HELP ANXIETY

Using essential oils in aromatherapy in conjunction with relaxation techniques can have an amazing effect on your mind and spirit. People with anxiety symptoms will find that essential oils with calming and soothing properties are among the best for tranquility in dealing with the wave of anxiety.

Certain essential oils can be used aromatically, while others can be applied topically or taken internally to encourage tranquility. When taken internally, these oils can help to calm the nervous system and promote relaxation. For example, Lavender oil can be used to ease feelings of tension. Similarly, Copaiba oil can be taken internally to help soothe and calm the nervous system. When using an essential oil topically, you will benefit from the aroma of the blend and the absorption through the skin. Essential oils can modulate the stress response and bring a calming effect to the body. Cypress, Cedarwood, Chamomile, Coriander, Ginger, and Frankincense, among others, have this effect.

Since everyone has different preferences and needs, each person will react differently to an essential oil and need to try other methods to determine which way suits them. This is why essential oils are especially good at promoting a restful environment, as you will find various methods and fragrances to suit your needs. If one approach doesn't create a relaxing atmosphere as you'd hoped, try another to see if it's a better fit for you.

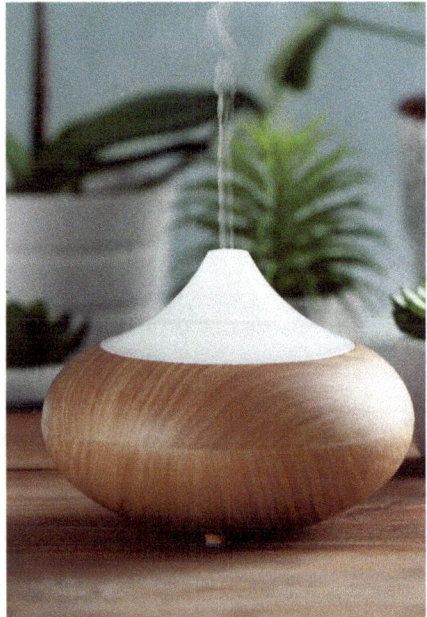

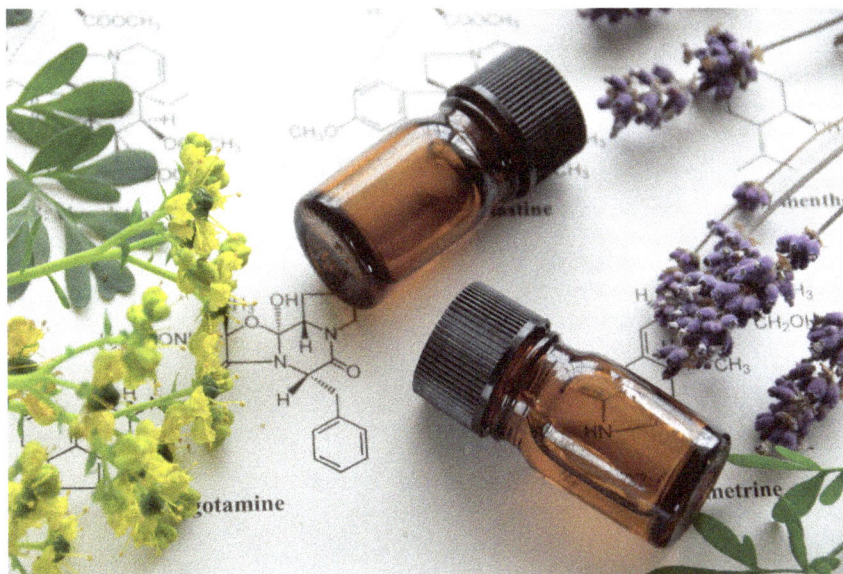

CHOOSING AN
ESSENTIAL OIL FOR ANXIETY

Educating yourself and learning about each essential oil's unique properties and benefits when choosing suitable oils for anxiety is important. The goal is to choose oils to help create a calm, tranquil, and relaxing environment. Luckily, there are dozens of essential oils with aromas that can promote a peaceful atmosphere.

Before choosing an essential oil for anxiety, you will want to consider its benefits, determined by its chemical components. Each essential oil has a unique chemical profile based on several factors, including the plant's part used for distillation and how it was distilled.

Depending on which plant part the oil is extracted from, some will have soothing properties, while others may be energizing and invigorating. Essential oils must have calming and soothing properties to be suitable for anxiety and produce a relaxed state. This will encourage your body to return to homeostasis.

You may have to experiment to see which oils work best for you when choosing essential oils for promoting calmness. Everyone has different preferences and needs, so what may work for one person may not work for you. This is what makes oil so unique in promoting a calming environment. If one essential oil doesn't produce the desired results, try another oil with similar components and see if it is a better fit.

Often memories associated with particular types of aromas may affect how the aroma will impact a person's emotional state. For instance, if you have a particularly strong emotional response to a particular oil or scent, it will affect its ability to influence your emotional well-being positively. If Cinnamon, usually a warm and comforting scent, has become associated with the death of a family member, you are less likely to be positively influenced by Cinnamon essential oil.

With time and practice, you will learn how your body and brain react to each essential oil. Try different oil combinations and various application methods to find which suits your need for promoting relaxation.

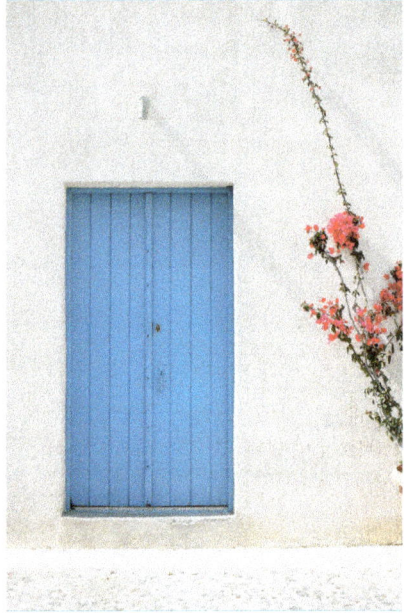

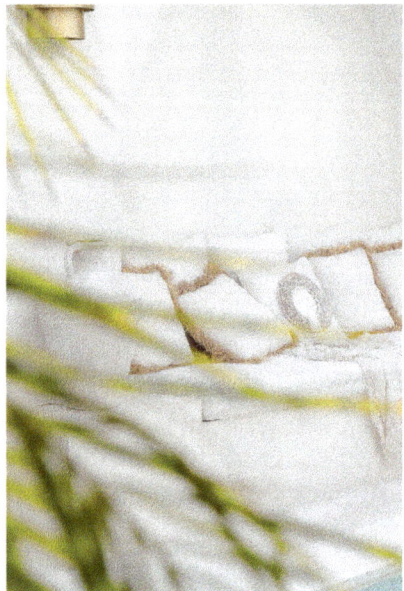

WHICH ESSENTIAL OILS ARE GOOD FOR ANXIETY?

It's important to educate yourself and learn about each essential oil's unique properties and benefits when trying to pick suitable oils for alleviating anxiety. The goal is to choose oils to help create a calm, tranquil, and relaxing environment. Luckily, there are dozens of essential oils with aromas that can promote a peaceful atmosphere.

Before choosing an essential oil for anxiety, you must first consider its benefits, which will depend on its chemical components. Each essential oil has a unique chemical profile from every other oil in its group based on several factors, including the plant's part used for distillation and how it was distilled.

Depending on the plant the oil is extracted from, some will have soothing properties, while others may be energizing and invigorating. An essential oil must have calming and soothing properties to be suitable for anxiety and produce a relaxed state. This is the perfect environment needed for tranquility.

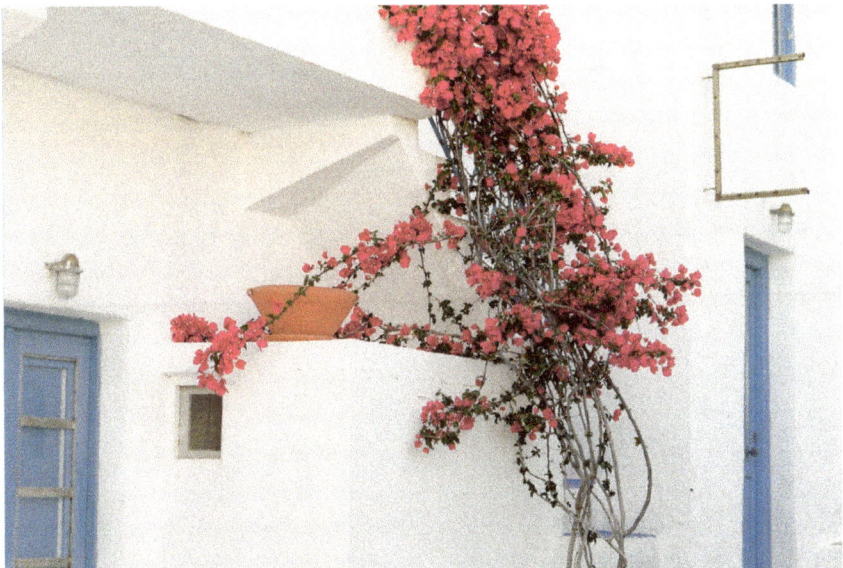

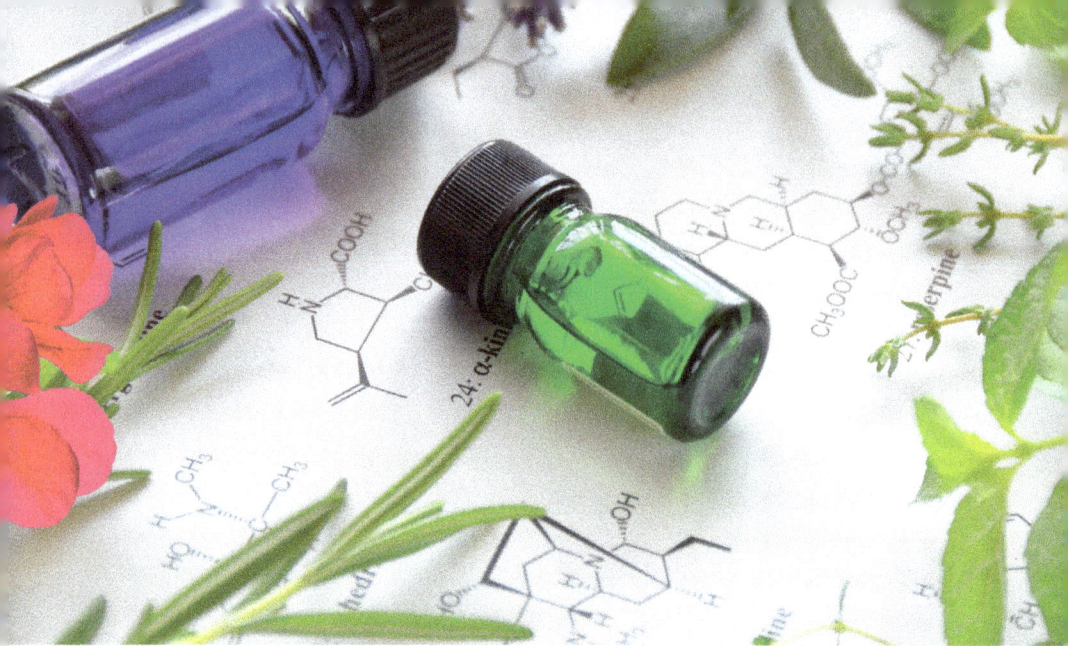

ESSENTIAL OIL PROPERTIES BENEFICIAL FOR ANXIETY

Let's look now at the properties that are beneficial for anxiety. Unique characteristics in an essential oil, such as warming, soothing, refreshing, and calming, will be the ones to look for when choosing an oil. Each oil is unique and contains a specific combination of chemical components. This means that one oil can have several valuable benefits.

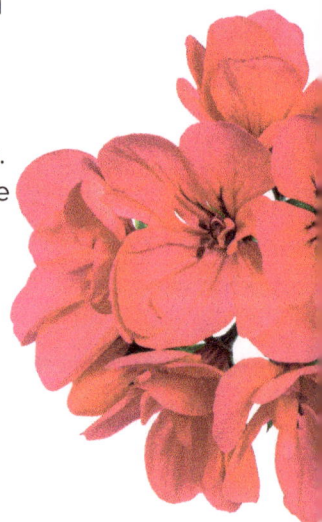

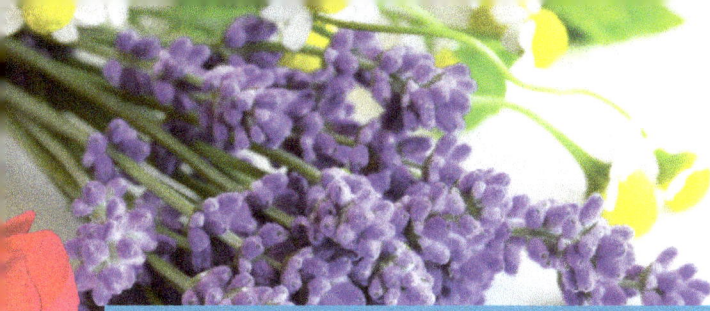

CALMING

Calming oils, consisting mainly of esters, can promote calm feelings for the body and mind. While the specific aromas listed below are very different, they produce similar effects on the body and can promote peaceful feelings and relax the mind. Many essential oils considered beneficial for anxiety possess calming therapeutic properties. Compounds like linalool and linalyl acetate, known for their relaxing properties, are abundant in essential oils like Lavender and Bergamot. These essential oils can be diffused to create a peaceful environment. They can also be taken internally to calm the nervous system, promote relaxation, and bring peace-of-mind.

ESSENTIAL OILS

- Lavender
- Clary Sage
- Petitgrain
- Roman Chamomile
- Bergamot
- Rose
- Orange
- Neroli
- Lemon
- Rose Geranium
- Birch
- Black Pepper
- Cassia
- Coriander
- Fennel
- Frankincense
- Geranium
- Jasmine
- Juniper Berry
- Melissa
- Oregano
- Patchouli
- Sandalwood
- Tangerine
- Vetiver
- Yarrow

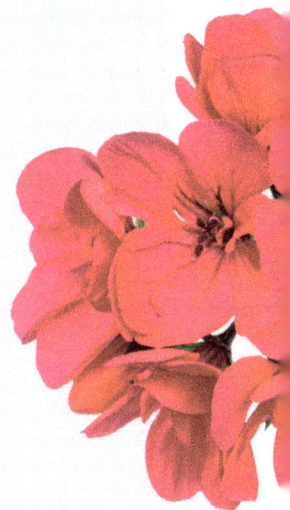

UPLIFTING

Uplifting oils will restore hope and inspiration and bring back optimism. Essential oils in this category are best used aromatically. These essential oils fight fatigue and help when you need a pick-me-up.

ESSENTIAL OILS

- Bergamot
- Cardamom
- Cedarwood
- Clary Sage
- Cypress
- Grapefruit
- Lemon
- Lime
- Melissa
- Sandalwood
- Tangerine
- Sweet Orange
- Ylang Ylang

REFRESHING

Refreshing oils can revitalize you and give you renewed strength. Try one of these oils to help with stimulation and pep. Use these oils aromatically or topically to revive the spirit.

ESSENTIAL OILS

- Cypress
- Geranium
- Grapefruit
- Lemon
- Lime
- Peppermint
- Sweet Orange
- Wintergreen

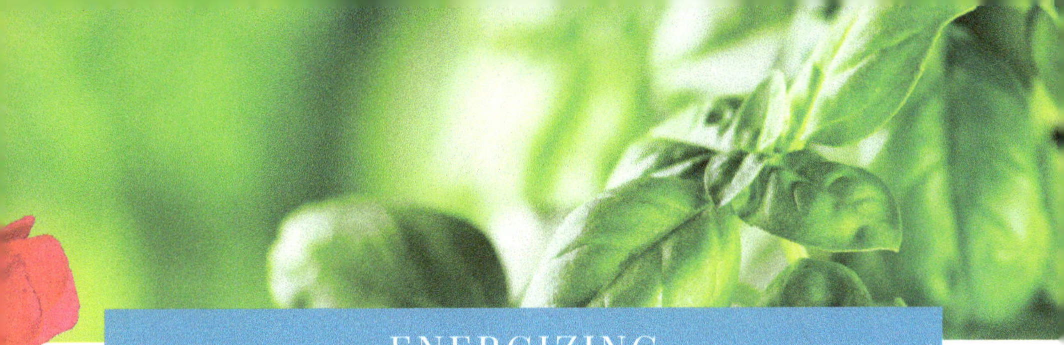

ENERGIZING

Oils in the energizing category can restore your strength and bring life back into you. Several essential oils contain properties that can uplift your mood, fight fatigue, and give you that extra boost of energy to get through the day. Try one or more of these oils to aid sluggishness and mental clarity.

ESSENTIAL OILS

- Basil
- Bergamot
- Clove
- Cypress
- Grapefruit
- Lemon
- Lemongrass
- Lime
- Rosemary
- Tangerine
- White Fir
- Sweet Orange

SOOTHING

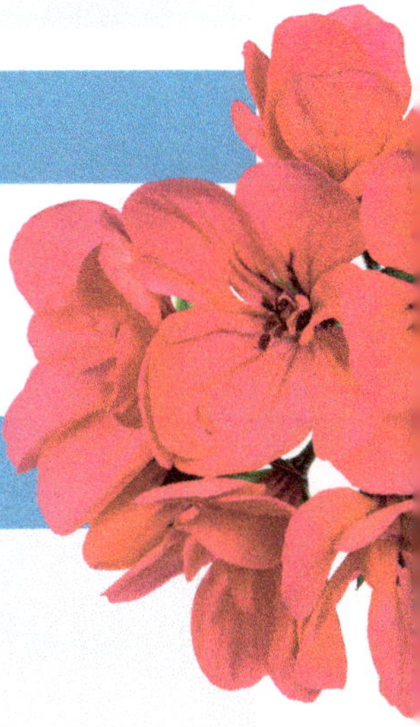

Oils in the soothing category can be applied topically or diffused aromatically to soothe the body and the mind.

ESSENTIAL OILS

- Melissa
- Ylang Ylang
- Dill

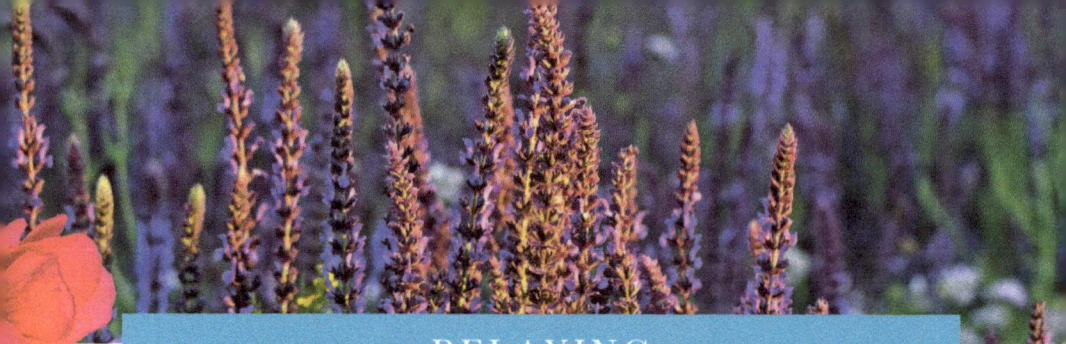

RELAXING

Oils in the relaxation category can be applied topically, diffused aromatically, and some ingested.

ESSENTIAL OILS

- Basil
- Cassia
- Cedarwood
- Clary Sage
- Cypress
- Fennel
- Geranium
- Jasmine
- Lavender
- Marjoram
- Myrrh
- Ravensara
- Roman Chamomile
- Vetiver
- White Fir
- Ylang Ylang

GROUNDING

Grounding oils are typically composed of alcohols or ketones and can help settle the body and mind by promoting calm feelings.

ESSENTIAL OILS

- Cedarwood
- Sandalwood
- Vetiver
- Spikenard
- Ylang Ylang
- Basil
- Clary Sage
- Cypress

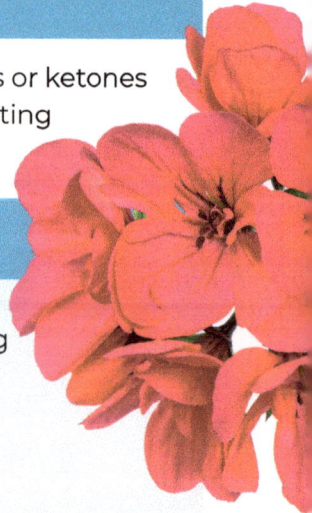

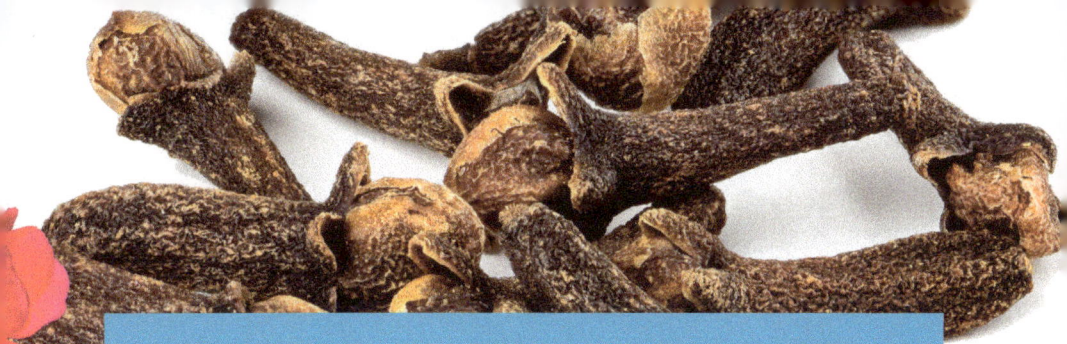

HARMONIZING

These essential oils promote harmony and balance to help the body and mind. Essential oils in this category are mainly composed of alcohols and help encourage serenity to help you relax.

ESSENTIAL OILS

- Cilantro
- Clary Sage
- Geranium
- Marjoram

WARMING

Warming oils can be used topically or aromatically to help promote calm, relaxed feelings. They often have a spicy aroma and feel warm on the skin. Remember to dilute warming oils before applying them to your skin, as they can be intense.

ESSENTIAL OILS

- Thyme
- Cassia
- Clove
- Cinnamon

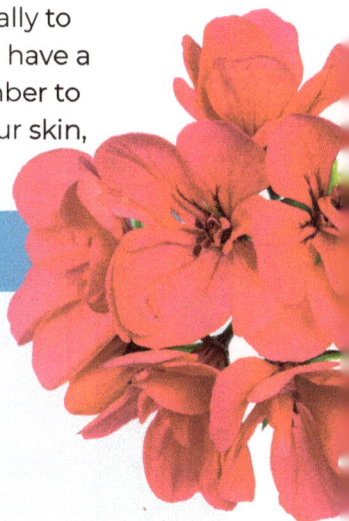

Be flexible and try different combinations to find which oils help you the most.

07
ESSENTIAL OILS
RECOMMENDED FOR ANXIETY

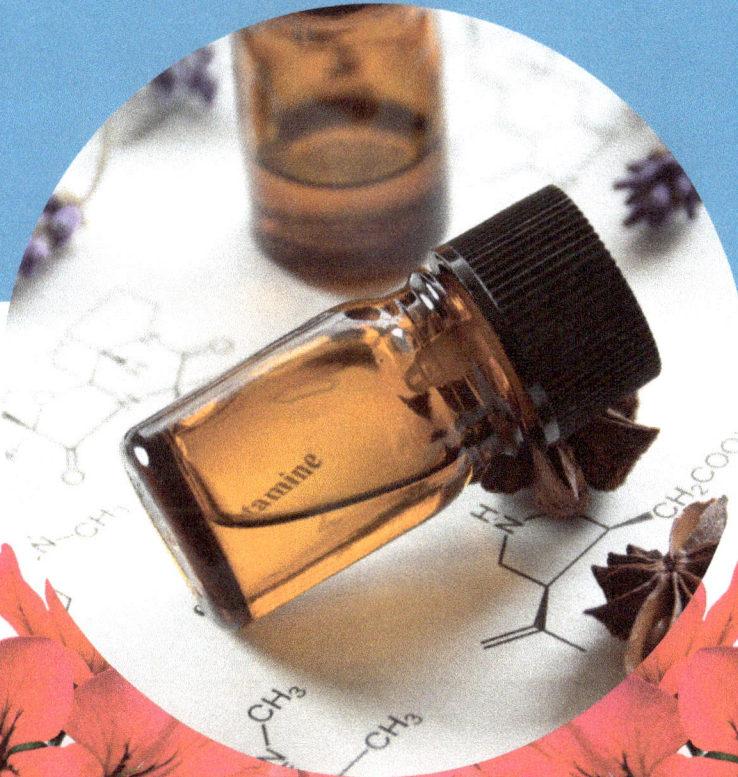

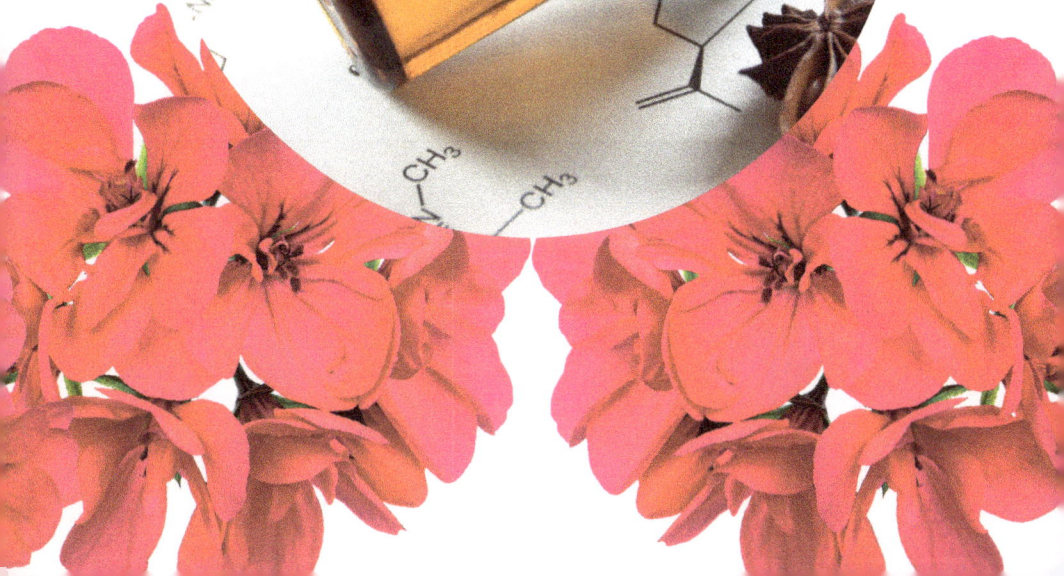

ESSENTIAL OILS FOR ANXIETY

If you are already familiar with essential oils, you probably know several oils that promote relaxation and may help you feel more grounded. Most essential oils smell nice, but the ones listed below are especially beneficial for anxiety.

Of course, essential oils are not a "magic pill." What may work for some people may be ineffective for you. This is because essential oils are adaptogens and affect people differently. Be flexible and try other oils until you find what works best.

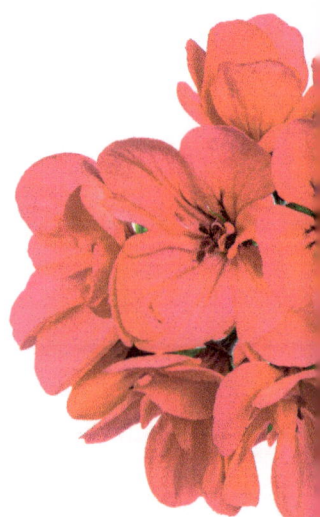

Basil relieves muscular aches, pains, mental fatigue, anxiety, and depression. It is incredibly soothing and uplifting and is popular with massage therapists for alleviating tension and stress in their patients. When applied in dilution, Basil is an excellent insect repellent as the linalool's mild analgesic properties are known to help relieve insect bites and stings. It is also highly effective as an antispasmodic, antiemetic, antiseptic, carminative, cephalic, expectorant, and immune support. This oil may irritate sensitive skin. A 2010 study published in *Phytomedicine* found that inhaling a mist containing linalool reversed anxiety symptoms in mice. A 2008 study published in Food Chemistry journal said that other chemicals in Basil had a synergistic effect on linalool, causing it to be soothing to the nervous system. Avoid use during pregnancy.

Usage: topical, inhalation
Note: top

BERGAMOT

Bergamot is a favorite oil for treating anxiety and depression. Studies have shown that Bergamot oil can reduce anxiety and improve the mood. The therapeutic properties of Bergamot include analgesic, antidepressant, antiseptic, antibiotic, antispasmodic, stomachic, calmative, cicatrisant, deodorant, digestive, febrifuge, vermifuge, and vulnerary. Unlike many other citrus oils that can be energizing, Bergamot is calming, reduces stress and anxiety, and possesses sedative qualities. It has been used for centuries to aid digestion and is thought to help maintain neural pathways in the brain. Research has also indicated that Bergamot can ease chronic pain, lowers the heart rate, and reduce blood pressure. It is helpful with anxiety and stress. Bergamot's sedative property helps the body relax and heal. Its antispasmodic property helps calm the muscles while increasing blood flow and circulation to promote a quicker healing time. Bergamot essential oil has phototoxic properties. Therefore, exposure to the sun must be avoided after use. It may also interfere with the activity of certain prescription drugs (NSAIDs, proton-pump inhibitors, acetaminophen, antiepileptics, immune modulators, blood-sugar medications, blood pressure medications, antidepressants, antipsychotics, diabetic medications, antihistamines, antibiotics, and anesthetics). While studies on Bergamot's capability to combat stress and anxiety are limited, studies do demonstrate Bergamot's ability to relax the mind, as shown in a 2017 study. Bergamot helps to level out emotions, discard negative emotions and fatigue, and reduce cortisol in saliva, as shown in a study published in 2015. A 2013 study in China found that patients were less anxious about upcoming surgery when they engaged in aromatherapy using Bergamot oil.

Usage: oral, topical, inhalation
Note: top

CEDARWOOD

Cedarwood is considered a natural sedative that can help reduce restlessness and anxiety. Cedarwood has a high content of sesquiterpenes, which promotes relaxation and prevents fatigue, a common side effect of stress. Studies have proven that Cedarwood is an excellent choice for improving one's night sleep with the help of the chemical called cedrol, which helps promote sleep by boosting parasympathetic activity and increasing serotonin production. Another study on hyperactive rats showed Cedarwood oil to have sedative properties and calmed the rats. Like Lavender, Cedarwood is considered suitable for clearing negative emotions. Because inhaling Cedarwood triggers the release of serotonin in the brain, which converts to melatonin, the essential oil is known for its sedative qualities and usefulness in treating insomnia. Cedarwood has been shown to decrease heart rate and blood pressure, maintaining its effectiveness in alleviating hypertension and anxiety. Cedarwood essential oil has also been found to reduce involuntary motor activity and prolong sleep for those people with restless legs and other movements during the night. It is considered a non-toxic and non-irritant oil. It is a relaxing and soothing oil that allows the brain to stop processing.

Usage: topical, inhalation
Note: base

German Chamomile is a relaxing and rejuvenating agent that calms nerves and reduces anxiety. German Chamomile is known for its anti-inflammatory abilities and can help alleviate muscle spasms and joint pain. Its therapeutic properties include analgesic, anti-allergic, anti-convulsive, antidepressant, antiseptic, antispasmodic, anti-inflammatory, cholagogue, diuretic, emmenagogue, febrifuge, hepatic, nervine, sedative, splenetic, stomachic, sudorific, tonic, vermifuge, and vasoconstrictor. Azulene gives this oil its intense blue color, while sesquiterpenes lend its calming effect. German Chamomile calms nerves, eases headaches, and aids in relaxation. It operates as a mild tranquilizer and as a sleep inducer. German Chamomile impacts the same areas of the brain and nervous system as popular anti-anxiety medications and can also assist in minimizing aches and pains. Its calming reputation and anxiety-reducing effects are due to apigenin, which German Chamomile contains and is known to bind to benzodiazepine receptors. Of course, the benefits of German Chamomile are not restricted to the use of its essential oil. The plant's flower can be enjoyed as a relaxing hot drink when brewed as a tea.

Usage: oral, topical, inhalation
Note: middle

Roman Chamomile is the most potent essential oil for battling anxiousness. Roman Chamomile is an ancient herb with therapeutic properties, including sedative and relaxing. It is recommended to treat insomnia, stress, restless leg syndrome, and nervous tension, so it is an excellent choice to help you relax and chill. Try combining Roman Chamomile essential oil with true Lavender essential oil for a more powerful treatment. The therapeutic properties of Roman Chamomile oil are analgesic, antispasmodic, antiseptic, antibiotic, anti-inflammatory, anti-infectious, antidepressant, antineuralgic, antiphlogistic, bactericidal, carminative, cholagogue, cicatrisant, emmenagogue, febrifuge, hepatic, sedative, nervine, digestive, tonic, sudorific, stomachic, vermifuge and vulnerary. It is non-toxic and non-irritating. Roman Chamomile's ability to act as a mild sedative to ease nerves and decrease anxiety to treat conditions like hysteria, nightmares, insomnia, and other sleep difficulties has also been researched. While the root of these effects is not determined, they appear to be psychological. Studies also have shown Roman Chamomile's effectiveness in relieving stress and anxiety. It has a warm, sweet, herbaceous scent that is relaxing and calming for both mind and body. Roman Chamomile's gentleness makes it especially valuable for restless children.

Usage: oral, topical, inhalation
Note: middle

Clary Sage can be used as an antidepressant and as a sedative. Women experiencing hormonal changes or menopause symptoms such as hot flashes find this oil beneficial. Clary Sage's properties are antidepressant, anticonvulsive, antispasmodic, anti-inflammatory, antiseptic, aphrodisiac, astringent, bactericidal, carminative, deodorant, digestive, emmenagogue, euphoric, hypotensive, nervine, sedative, stomachic, uterine, and nerve tonic. Clary Sage oil is non-toxic and non-sensitizing. Its anti-inflammatory and antispasmodic properties help to calm and soothe the body and mind. It also aids in reducing pain associated with inflammation. Clary Sage is a natural sedative that may reduce your cortisol levels, known as the stress hormone. Do not use it during pregnancy or if you are at risk for breast cancer, as it may have an estrogen-like effect on the body. Clary Sage is similar to Valerian in that it affects the GABA receptors, which help reduce anxiety. Clary Sage also has mood-lifting properties that are useful in treating patients who suffer from depression.

Usage: oral, topical, inhalation
Note: top-middle

CORIANDER

Coriander works as an analgesic, antirheumatic, antispasmodic, carminative, deodorant, fungicidal, revitalizing, and stimulating. It relieves mental fatigue, migraine pain, stress, and nervous debility. Coriander's warming effect helps alleviate pain such as rheumatism, arthritis, and muscle spasms. The healing properties of Cilantro or Coriander oil are attributed to phytonutrient content, including carvone, geraniol, limonene, borneol, camphor, elemol, and linalool. Coriander is traditionally used in India for its anti-inflammatory properties. Coriander oil is also beneficial for removing heavy metals and toxins from the body.

Usage: oral, topical, inhalation
Note: top

CYPRESS

Cypress is an incredibly gentle oil that calms and soothes anxiousness while positively affecting one's mood. It assists with varicose veins and bodily fluids by improving circulation. Its properties include antibacterial, anti-infectious, anti-inflammatory, anti-rheumatic, antiseptic, antispasmodic, astringent, decongestant, diuretic, and vein tonic. Avoid use during pregnancy. It may interact with aspirin, blood pressure, antiplatelet, and anticoagulant medications.

Usage: topical, inhalation
Note: middle-base

DILL

Dill is a stimulating, revitalizing, restoring, purifying, and balancing oil. Dill oil, when used aromatically, can help lessen stress and reduce anxious feelings. This oil can be used internally before bed to help promote restful sleep. Its healing properties include antispasmodic, carminative, digestive, disinfectant, galactagogue, sedative, stomachic and sudorific. Dill helps relieve cramps, diarrhea, flatulence, and indigestion. Dill Seed is non-toxic and non-irritating. Avoid use during pregnancy.

Usage: oral, topical, inhalation
Note: middle

FRANKINCENSE

Frankincense is very soothing and has been the subject of multiple studies for its anxiolytic properties that help reduce anxiety. Frankincense reduces inflammation's pain while calming the body and mind and promoting healing. The therapeutic properties of Frankincense oil are antiseptic, astringent, antirheumatic, antispasmodic, carminative, cicatrisant, cytophylactic, digestive, diuretic, emmenagogue, expectorant, sedative, tonic, uterine and vulnerary. Frankincense causes relaxation and sends messages to the limbic system that help reduce stress and improve mood. Frankincense essential oil helps open passageways, which can help reduce snoring and allow your body to take deep, calming breaths. This oil is non-toxic, non-irritating, and non-sensitizing.

Usage: oral, topical, inhalation
Note: base

GERANIUM

Geranium is excellent for helping improve the emotional aspect of life and uplifting mood. Geranium is well tolerated by most individuals and helps balance the hormonal system. Research published in 2015 showed that Geranium reduces anxiety in pregnant women during labor. The study on 100 women showed how Geranium effectively relieves stress during pregnancy and reduces diastolic blood pressure after inhaling Geranium essential oil.

Usage: oral, topical, inhalation
Note: base

JASMINE

Jasmine is well respected for its aphrodisiac properties and is a sensual, soothing, calming oil that promotes love and peace. In a 2010 study, Jasmine was as effective for calming nerves as a sleeping pill or sedative drug, except without side effects. It is important to note that all absolutes are extremely concentrated by nature. The complexity of the fragrance, particularly the rare and exotic notes, is well regarded as an aphrodisiac. However, it is also considered an antidepressant, antiseptic, cicatrisant, expectorant, galactagogue, parturient, sedative, uterine and antispasmodic. Jasmine has been known to assist with restless sleep, enhancing sleep quality. Avoid use during the first and second trimesters of pregnancy.

Usage: topical, inhalation
Note: base

LAVENDER

Lavender is an effective essential oil predominately made up of alcohols and esters and has several therapeutic properties, many associated with relaxation. Lavender is the most popular essential oil, but be aware that several species, such as Spike Lavender (Lavandula latifolia) and the hybrid Lavandin (Lavandula x intermedia), have very similar properties but are not as sedating as true Lavender. Lavender is known to improve sleep quality, increase the time spent in deep, slow-wave sleep, and relieve restlessness and negative emotions. Lavender is known to calm anxiety and offers sedative effects. Research revealed that a Lavender foot bath could improve blood flow and encourage changes in the autonomic nervous system often seen when people are relaxed. Lavender essential oil is an excellent choice for its ability to help relax the body and help reduce insomnia caused by anxiety and stress. One study published in *The Journal of Alternative and Complementary Medicine* used a memory test with the aroma of Lavender to see how participants performed the analysis while stressed. Those who inhaled Lavender performed superior to those who inhaled a placebo aroma. Research published in 2013 has shown that a 3% Lavender oil spray on clothes reduced work-related stress for three to four days; this proves how powerful Lavender is in relieving stress, even with just 3% of the actual oil being used. Lavender has been shown in a study to help ease anxiety and stress-related disorders (ex., PTSD) and help relax the brain. The therapeutic properties of Lavender essential oil are antiseptic, analgesic, anticonvulsant, antidepressant, anti-rheumatic, antispasmodic, anti-inflammatory, antiviral, bactericide, carminative, cholagogue, cicatrisant, cordial, cytophylactic, decongestant, deodorant, diuretic, emmenagogue, hypotensive, nervine, rubefacient, sedative, sudorific and vulnerary. Lavender is non-toxic, non-irritating, and non-sensitizing. Do not use it during the first trimester of pregnancy.

Usage: oral, topical, inhalation
Note: middle

LAVANDIN

Lavandin properties include analgesic, anticonvulsive, antidepressant, antiphlogistic, antirheumatic, antiseptic, antispasmodic, antiviral, bactericidal, carminative, cholagogue, cicatrisant, cordial, cytophylactic, decongestant, deodorant, and diuretic. It is considered one of the most valuable and versatile essential oils, from easing sore muscles and joints, relieving muscle stiffness, clearing the lungs and sinuses from phlegm to healing wounds and dermatitis. Its analgesic properties aid in alleviating pain. Its calming scent reduces anxiety and promotes sleep. This oil is non-toxic, non-irritating, and non-sensitizing. Use caution during pregnancy.

Usage: topical, inhalation
Note: middle

LEMON

Lemon is uplifting and energizing with its refreshing and cooling properties. Lemon also possesses a chemical called linalool, which is known to help with stress, boost sleep, and even have antidepressant properties. Lemon also contains antidepressant-like and anxiolytic properties known to reduce anxiety and tension within the body, as shown in a study published in 2006. According to a 2011 study conducted in Brazil, essential oils from the leaves of the Lemon plant have the rare quality of decreasing symptoms of anxiety and depression. This study, conducted on mice, involved the oral application of essential oils. It is suitable for the circulatory system and aids blood flow, reducing blood pressure. Citral, myrcene, and limonene, all present in citrus oils, have been shown in some studies to lengthen sleep duration and relax muscles. Lemon's therapeutic properties are anti-anemic, antimicrobial, anti-rheumatic, anti-sclerotic, antiseptic, bactericidal, carminative, cicatrisant, depurative, diaphoretic, diuretic, febrifuge, hemostatic, hypotensive, insecticidal, rubefacient, tonic and vermifuge. Lemon is non-toxic but could cause skin irritation for some. Check for phototoxicity before exposure to direct sunlight.

Usage: oral, topical, inhalation
Note: top

LEMONGRASS

Lemongrass essential oil is known for its stimulating qualities and makes an excellent antidepressant. This essential oil promotes blood circulation by dilating the blood vessels, allowing uninterrupted blood flow. Lemongrass helps reduce inflammation. Lemongrass not only tones but fortifies the nervous system and can be used in the bath for soothing muscular nerves and pain with its potent analgesic and anti-inflammatory qualities. This oil relieves the symptoms of jet lag, helps with nervousness and anxiety, and clears headaches. The therapeutic properties of Lemongrass oil are analgesic, antidepressant, antimicrobial, antipyretic, antiseptic, astringent, bactericidal, carminative, deodorant, diuretic, febrifuge, fungicidal, galactagogue, insecticidal, nervine, nervous system sedative and tonic. Avoid use with individuals with glaucoma. Use caution in prostatic hyperplasia and with skin hypersensitivity or damaged skin. Safe for topical and ingestion if appropriately diluted. It can be used topically, through diffusion/inhalation, and internally. A 2011 article published in *The Journal of Ethnopharmacology* found that Lemongrass essential oil decreased symptoms of stress in mice. In another study published in *Phytomedicine*, a tea made with Lemongrass had a calming impact on subjects.

Usage: oral, topical, inhalation
Note: top

MANDARIN

Mandarin is often used to ease anxiety and as a digestive aid. This tangy oil increases circulation to the skin and reduces fluid retention. Mandarin therapeutic properties include antiseptic, antispasmodic, cytophylactic, depurative, sedative, stomachic, and tonic. Direct sunlight should be avoided after use, as it may be phototoxic.

Usage: oral, topical, inhalation
Note: top

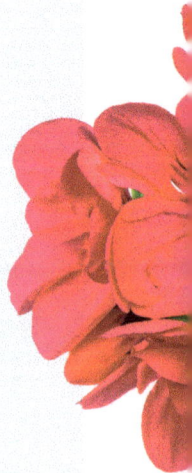

Marjoram essential oil helps with insomnia due to its calming and sedating action on the nervous system. Marjoram is thought to increase alertness and focus while reducing chronic stress. It lowers blood pressure, eases nervousness and hyperactivity, and soothes loneliness, grief, and rejection. Sweet Marjoram's sleep-inducing effects are thought to be even more effective than those of Lavender and Chamomile; both are used more often as sleep aids. Marjoram is a comforting oil that can be massaged into the affected area or added to a warm compress to ease discomfort. Marjoram's pain-relieving properties are helpful for rheumatic pains, sprains, spasms, swollen joints, and achy muscles. Marjoram is a great relaxant beneficial for headaches, migraines, and insomnia. Marjoram's therapeutic properties are analgesic, antispasmodic, antiarthritic, antirheumatic, anaphrodisiac, antiseptic, antiviral, anti-inflammatory, bactericidal, carminative, cephalic, cordial, diaphoretic, digestive, diuretic, emmenagogue, expectorant, fungicidal, hypotensive, laxative, nervine, sedative, stomachic, vasodilator, and vulnerary. Its sedative properties allow the body to heal, reduce inflammation and eliminate pain. Marjoram is generally non-toxic, non-irritating, and non-sensitizing.

Usage: oral, topical, inhalation
Note: middle

MELISSA

Melissa, also called Lemon Balm, is well known for its antidepressant and uplifting properties. Its healing properties include being antidepressant, anti-inflammatory, antiviral, antispasmodic, bactericidal, carminative, cordial, diaphoretic, emmenagogue, nervine, sedative, stomachic, sudorific, and tonic. Melissa has strong sedative qualities and treats emotional trauma and shock. It is considered non-sensitizing and non-toxic. Please check with your healthcare provider before use during pregnancy.

Usage: oral, topical, inhalation
Note: middle-top

NEROLI

Neroli is used for its relaxing and slightly hypnotic effects, and it can also help with lucid dreaming and spark creativity. It aids sleep due to its soothing qualities and functionality as a natural tranquilizer. One study found that Neroli oil, in combination with Lavender and Chamomile oil, was effective in reducing anxiety, increasing sleep, and stabilizing blood pressure. Another study revealed that Neroli could reduce postmenopausal symptoms, increase sexual desire, and reduce blood pressure in postmenopausal women. Neroli is also known to help relieve muscle spasms and heart palpitations. Neroli's therapeutic properties are antidepressant, antiseptic, anti-infectious, antispasmodic, aphrodisiac, bactericidal, carminative, cicatrisant, cytophylactic, cordial, deodorant, digestive, sedative, and tonic. This oil is non-toxic and non-sensitizing.

Usage: topical, inhalation
Note: middle-top

OPOPONAX

Opoponax, also known as Sweet Myrrh, properties include analgesic, antifungal, anti-anxiety, antibacterial, anti-inflammatory, antiseptic, astringent, antispasmodic, calming, and carminative, disinfectant, emmenagogue, expectorant, immune stimulant, stomachic, sedative, tonic, and vulnerary. This oil is helpful for menopause. Topically this oil may be used similarly to Myrrh in balms, ointments, and salves. It is also beneficial for relaxing muscles, reducing stress, and treating anxiety. It may be phototoxic; therefore, avoid direct sunlight for 12 hours. Avoid use during pregnancy.

Usage: topical, inhalation
Note: base

ORANGE

Orange essential oil has been shown to reduce acute anxiety and improve mood. A 2018 study in Brazil found that mice exposed to Orange essential oils as a mist in the atmosphere showed more social tendencies than a control group. This study suggests that Orange essential oil, especially in aerosol form, may decrease symptoms of anxiety and depression. In another study, Sweet Orange diffused through a mister calmed study participants better than a control group, according to a 2012 study published in *The Journal of Alternative and Complementary Medicine.*

Usage: oral, topical, inhalation
Note: top

PATCHOULI

Patchouli is beneficial for combating nervous disorders and nausea, treating depression, and reducing fever. This oil's therapeutic properties include antidepressant, anti-inflammatory, antimicrobial, antiseptic, antitoxic, antiviral, aphrodisiac, astringent, bactericidal, deodorant, diuretic, fungicidal, nervine, prophylactic, stimulating, and tonic agent. As a sedative oil, it allows the body to relax and rest, allowing healing to begin. It may interact with aspirin, blood pressure, antiplatelet, and anticoagulant medications and increase the risk of bleeding among people with bleeding disorders.

Usage: oral, topical, inhalation
Note: base

PETITGRAIN

Petitgrain is believed to have uplifting properties and is used for calming anger and stress. Petitgrain is valued for its ability to reduce pain and spasms in the lower intestines. Its calming qualities make it a favorite for insomnia. This oil's properties include antidepressant, antiseptic, antispasmodic, deodorant, immuno-support and stimulant, tonic, and sedative for the nervous system. Petitgrain is generally considered non-toxic, non-irritating, and non-sensitizing.

Usage: oral, topical, inhalation
Note: top

ROSALINA

Rosalina is well known for its antiseptic, spasmolytic, and anticonvulsant properties. Rosalina helps to relax and calm individuals who may be stressed deeply. It is helpful for insomnia and other sleep disorders. Rosalina's therapeutic properties include antibacterial, antimicrobial, analgesic, anti-anxiety, cicatrisant, immunostimulant, antiviral, anti-inflammatory, and mucolytic. Avoid use during pregnancy.

Usage: topical, inhalation
Note: middle

ROSE GERANIUM

Rose Geranium has the ability to both uplift and sedate. It is considered a wonder oil for emotions and balances the hormonal system. Rose Geranium is non-toxic, non-irritant, and generally non-sensitizing, though it can cause sensitivity in some people. Its therapeutic properties include antidepressant, anti-inflammatory, antiseptic, astringent, antispasmodic, cicatrisant, emmenagogue, and sedative. Avoid use during pregnancy.

Usage: oral, topical, inhalation
Note: middle

Rose is an uplifting aphrodisiac and is excellent for meditation. Rose essential oil treats depression, grief, anger, and other unpleasant emotions. It supports the heart and is considered one of the most amazing remedies for female problems, such as balancing hormones during menopause. It helps to reduce muscle spasms and pain from injury and inflammation. The therapeutic properties of Rose are antidepressant, antiphlogistic, antiseptic, antispasmodic, antiviral, aphrodisiac, astringent, bactericidal, choleretic, cicatrisant, depurative, emmenagogue, hemostatic, hepatic, laxative, nervous system sedative, stomachic and a tonic for the heart, liver, stomach, and uterus. Rose oil relieves pain by activating the TRPV1 receptor (a sensor that detects pain). Avoid use during the first trimester of pregnancy.

Usage: oral, topical, inhalation
Note: base

ROSEWOOD

Rosewood is credited as being a bactericidal, antifungal, antiviral, antiseptic, antispasmodic, anti-parasitic, cellular stimulant, immune system stimulant, tissue regenerator, tonic, antidepressant, antimicrobial, analgesic, cephalic, sedative, and an aphrodisiac. It is also regarded as a general balancer of emotions and helps with insomnia. Rosewood is rich in linalool, a chemical that can be transformed into several derivatives of value to the flavor and fragrance industries. It is a possible irritant to sensitive skin. Avoid use during pregnancy.

Usage: topical, inhalation
Note: base

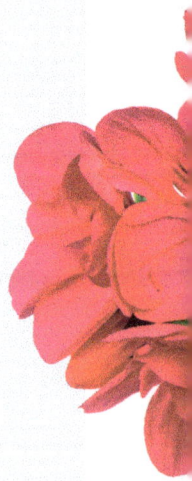

SANDALWOOD

Sandalwood is known to create an exotic, sensual mood with a reputation as an aphrodisiac. Aromatherapy has been used for years to reduce and relieve inflammation. Sandalwood reduces swelling and muscle spasms by inhibiting the 5-lipoxygenase (5-LOX) enzyme in the inflammation response. Its sedative effect allows the body to relax and heal. Sandalwood is used to help combat mood disturbances and stress. Santalol, a major component of Sandalwood oil, has been found to have a depressive effect on the central nervous system, enabling users to get more sleep. Sandalwood's therapeutic properties are antiphlogistic, antiseptic, antispasmodic, astringent, carminative, diuretic, emollient, expectorant, sedative, and tonic. Sandalwood can aid in relaxation and calm anxiety. It is also known to have sedative effects. Sandalwood is considered non-toxic, non-irritant, and non-sensitizing.

Usage: oral, topical, inhalation
Note: base

SPEARMINT

Spearmint essential oil is known for calming nausea and combating headaches. It is an uplifting oil, making it ideal for alleviating fatigue and depression. This is best taken directly for acute symptoms: try sniffing the oil from a bottle or rubbing a small amount on your forehead.

Usage: oral, topical, inhalation
Note: middle

SPIKENARD

Spikenard is used for rashes, wrinkles, cuts, insomnia, migraines, and wounds. It brings peaceful tranquility. This oil's therapeutic properties are anti-inflammatory, antifungal, antispasmodic, sedative and tonic. Spikenard should be avoided during pregnancy.

Usage: oral, topical, inhalation
Note: base

VALERIAN

Valerian is used in combating nervousness, restlessness, tension, agitation, panic attacks, and headaches resulting from nervous tension. It has also been used on muscle spasms, heart palpitations, cardiovascular spasms, and neuralgia. Valerian is a suitable replacement for catnip based on similar chemical components and is gaining popularity as a natural alternative to commercially available sedatives. The therapeutic properties of Valerian are antispasmodic, bactericidal, carminative, diuretic, hypnotic, hypotensive, regulator, sedative, and stomachic. It has possible skin-sensitizing properties, though it is non-toxic and non-irritating at low doses. Valerian has been shown to reduce anxiety, which can help you to fall asleep and stay asleep longer and improve the quality of your sleep. It is calming to the nervous system and helps with restlessness. Avoid use during pregnancy and with children.

Usage: oral, topical, inhalation
Note: base

VETIVER

Vetiver is profoundly relaxing and comforting. Its calming and soothing effect helps to relieve and reduce symptoms of inflammation. It helps to promote circulation and reduce pain. This oil helps dispel irritability, anger, and hysteria while balancing the hormonal system. It is relaxing to the nervous system and helps with overstimulation. Vetiver oil's therapeutic properties are antiseptic, aphrodisiac, cicatrisant, nervine, sedative, tonic, and vulnerary. There is no known toxicity.

Usage: oral, topical, inhalation
Note: base

YLANG YLANG

Ylang Ylang assists with problems such as high blood pressure, rapid breathing, heartbeat, nervous conditions, impotence, and frigidity. The therapeutic properties of Ylang Ylang are antidepressant, antiseborrheic, antiseptic, aphrodisiac, hypotensive, nervine, and sedative. Ylang Ylang helps balance both sides of the brain and aid in the processing and releasing negative emotions like anger. Ylang Ylang oil can be combined with Bergamot oil to help reduce blood pressure, pulse, stress, anxiety, and cortisol. When it comes to sleep, Ylang Ylang can help you fall asleep faster while lowering stress and anxiety. Ylang Ylang is also a sedative and can have calming effects in relieving anxiety. Ylang Ylang may cause sensitivity in some people, and excessive use may lead to headaches and nausea. This oil is not recommended if you have low blood pressure. Ylang Ylang is an excellent oil for falling asleep if you find your mind racing from the day's activities and struggle to settle it.

Usage: oral, topical, inhalation
Note: base

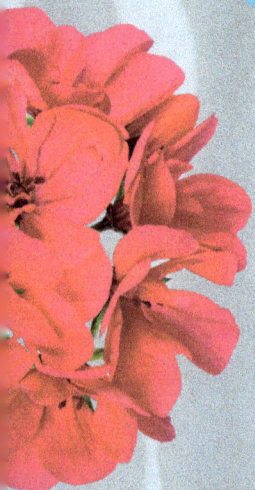

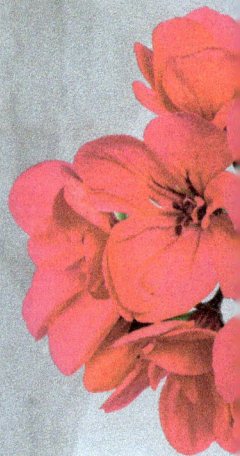

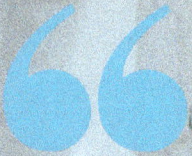

> *A massage oil blend with 10-15% essential oil and 85-90% carrier oil will ensure a powerful massage oil that is smooth and great-smelling.*

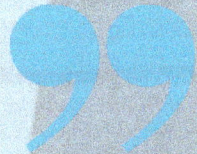

08 / CARRIER OILS

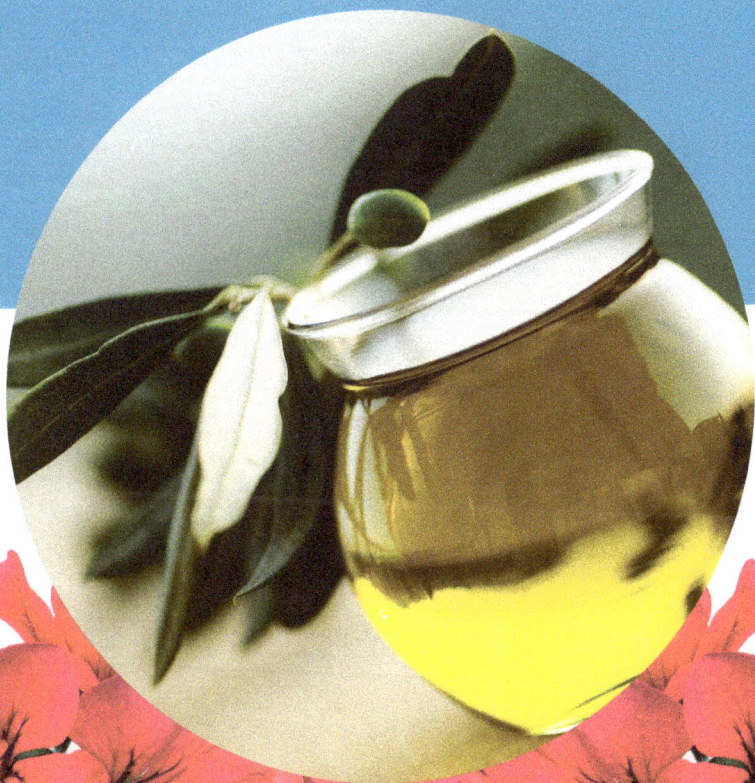
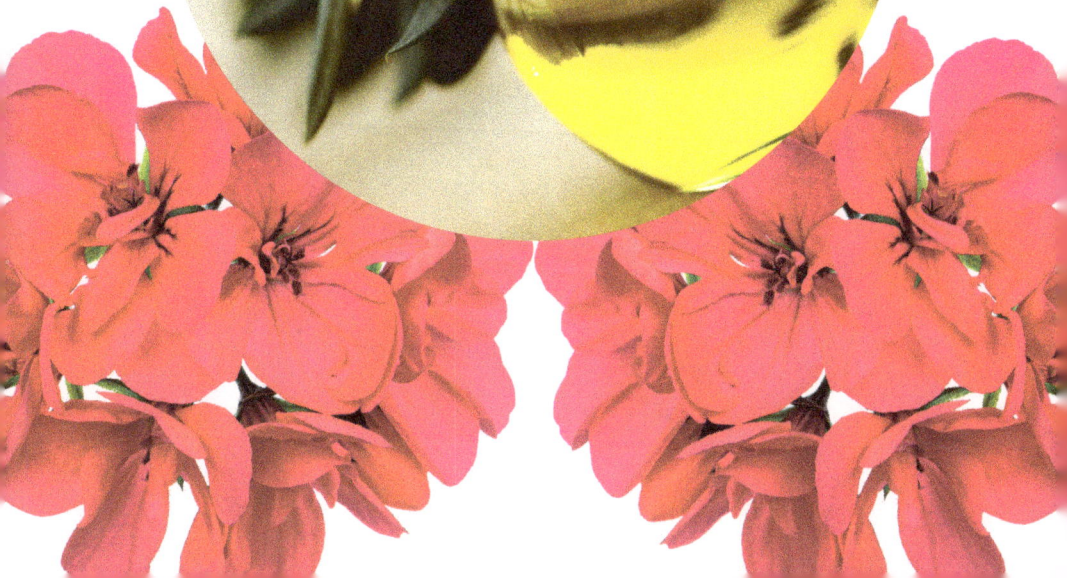

When you use essential oils topically, you will want to dilute them with a carrier or vegetable oil. Carrier and infused oils are used to dilute essential oils and absolutes by offering the necessary lubrication and moisture to the skin for aromatherapy.

Carrier oils come from nuts, seeds, or kernels that contain essential fatty acids, fat-soluble vitamins, minerals, and other crucial nutrients. You will find a variety of carrier oils to choose from, each possessing different therapeutic properties.

Distinct from essential oils, carrier oils do not contain aromatic scents (or only a very faint scent) and evaporate due to their large molecular structure. For this reason, most consider carrier oils just a vehicle for applying essential oils to the skin in massage. However, they offer healing properties that essential oils do not possess. Your aromatherapy experience can be significantly enhanced by choosing the best combination of carrier and essential oils.

The dilution of essential oils is always recommended because of their potency. Some can be harmful in large doses to some sensitive groups. One should exercise caution when dealing with oils such as Oregano, Cinnamon Bark/Leaf, and Cassia.

Carrier oils are used to dilute essential oil blends and are the main component when making essential oil blends.

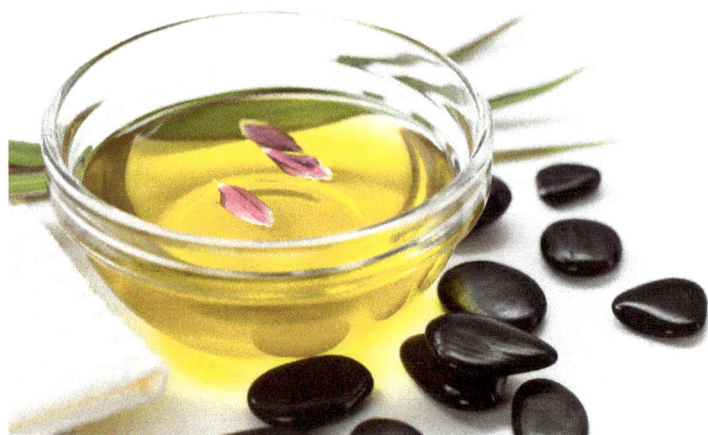

SHELF LIFE OF CARRIER OILS

A carrier oil's shelf life, the length of time before a particular oil begins to turn rancid, can be significantly influenced by heat and light.

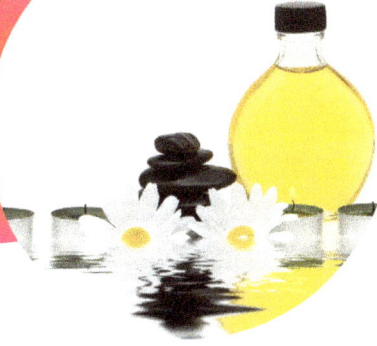

You will want to store your oils in a cool, dark place to preserve their freshness and, in some cases, refrigerate, as heat and sunlight can shorten their shelf life. When refrigerating, oils may appear cloudy but will regain their transparency upon returning to room temperature. If you have a large amount of carrier oil, you can freeze the unused portion until ready for use.

When carrier oils are used with essential oils topically, they provide a mechanism for the volatile oils to be transported more effectively. Most essential oils, when applied externally, move through the body system in an hour. A carrier oil, thicker than a volatile oil, "holds" the essential oil in place, delivering longer-lasting healing.

Essential oils in aromatherapy are highly concentrated and potent. Although there are only a few exceptions to using essential oils "neat" or undiluted (such as Lavender and Chamomile), it is ideal always to use a carrier oil with your essential oils to avoid having an adverse effect or skin irritation.

CARRIER OIL	SHELF LIFE
Almond (sweet)	12 months
Apricot Kernel	6-12 months
Argan	24 months
Avocado	12 months
Borage	6 months
Carrot Seed	12 months
Cocoa Butter	3-5 years
Coconut (fractionated)	Indefinite
Coconut (virgin)	2-4 years
Evening Primrose	6-12 months
Grapeseed	3-6 months
Hemp Seed	12 months
Jojoba	Indefinite
Olive	12-18 months
Safflower	24 months
Shea Butter	Indefinite
Walnut	12 months

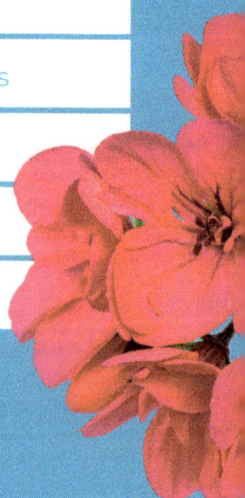

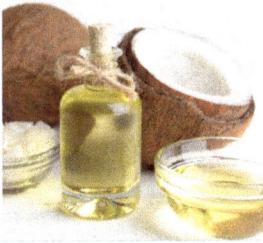

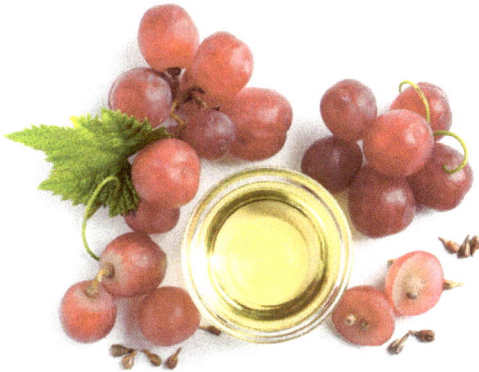

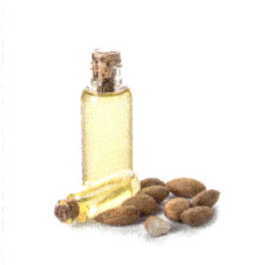

Carrier oils provide the much-needed lubrication, allowing hands to move freely over the skin, and helping with the absorption of essential oils into the body. Choose a carrier oil that is light, non-sticky, and can effectively penetrate the skin. Always check the label to ensure it's 100% pure, unrefined, and cold-pressed.

TIP: Try not to mix too much of your favorite massage blend in advance if you don't use it immediately.

With the vast selection of carrier oils, each with various therapeutic benefits, choosing one will depend on the area it's being applied to, the treatment plan, and any skin sensitivities. When using oil for massage, viscosity is an important consideration. Some carrier oils may work better than others in specific applications. For example, Grapeseed oil is generally very thin, while Olive oil is much thicker, and others, such as Sunflower and Sweet Almond, have viscosities halfway between these extremes. You can easily blend carrier oils to combine viscosity properties, absorption rate, and benefits.

TIP: When shopping for a good quality carrier oil, make sure it's cold-pressed to retain all its natural qualities.

ALMOND OIL

Almond Oil is one of the most useful, practical, and moderately priced carrier oils. It is ideal for all skin types as it moisturizes and reconditions the skin with its satiny smooth texture. This pale-yellow oil quickly absorbs into the skin, leaving your skin feeling soft and non-greasy. Sweet Almond relieves itching, soreness, dryness, and inflammation and is especially beneficial for eczema. As a lightly nutty refined oil rich in fatty acids, proteins, and vitamin D, it is everyone's favorite massage base oil for loosening stiff muscles and achy joints.

Dilution: Can be used at 100%.

COCONUT OIL

Coconut Oil (Fractionated) seems to be quickly becoming the carrier oil of choice because of its broad use in alternative medicine and healing. While it is fractionated, no change has been made chemically. Instead, its molecular structure "fraction" has been separated, allowing it to remain liquid at room temperature, making it much more helpful in aromatherapy. Coconut oil is a moisturizer for the body that delivers many health benefits. Its light, easily absorbable texture gives skin a smooth satin effect with virtually no scent of its own and indefinite shelf life.

Dilution: Can be used at 100%.

COCONUT OIL

Coconut Oil (Virgin) has an incredible balance of natural saturated fatty acids with antibacterial and antiviral properties not found in other oils. Coconut oil is perfect as a skin conditioner for nearly all skin conditions and is believed to stimulate hair growth. It has a light, aromatic coconut scent that becomes solid at room temperature. For this reason, blending with other carrier oils in your body care products is recommended. It is fully digestible and is considered a healthy cooking oil. Several virgin coconut oils are high in antioxidants, positively associated with reducing oxidative stress and thus lowering blood pressure.

Dilution: It can be used alone directly, but it is recommended to use 10-25% dilution with other carrier oils.

GRAPESEED OIL

Grapeseed Oil is a lovely, light green, and odorless oil used as a base oil for many creams, lotions, and carrier oil. Grapeseed oil is pressed from the seeds of a grape and contains OPCs, flavonoids, vitamin E, resveratrol, and fatty acids. It is non-allergenic and has very high levels of linoleic acid, with traces of proanthocyanidins, which are very potent antioxidants. It is especially beneficial for all skin types because of its natural non-allergenic properties. Grapeseed works well, especially when other oils do not absorb well, without leaving a greasy feeling after application. Grapeseed makes an ideal carrier oil for body massage bases. Saturation takes longer than some other carrier oils.

Dilution: Can be used at 100%.

JOJOBA OIL

Jojoba Oil is bright and golden in color and is known as one of the best oils (actually a liquid wax) for hair and skin. It penetrates the skin quickly and is excellent for nourishing and healing inflamed skin, psoriasis, eczema, or dermatitis. It is suitable for all skin types and promotes a healthy, glowing complexion by gently unclogging the pores and lifting embedded impurities. Jojoba is suitable for all aromatherapy uses other than a full-body massage. And, because of the oil's antioxidants, it does not become rancid and can even prevent rancidity in other oils.

Dilution: It can be used at 100%, but many use a 10% dilution with other carrier oils due to its price.

OLIVE OIL

Olive Oil (Extra Virgin) is light to medium green in color with a slightly dense texture. It is very soothing and carries disinfecting and healing properties. Olive oil is legendary since it has been used over the centuries for multiple purposes, but due to its overpowering scent, this oil does not work well for massages. However, it is beneficial in some lotions for burns or scars. Olive is accommodating for dry, damaged, or split hair and is soothing for inflamed skin such as eczema. The "virgin" indicates it comes from the first pressing of the fruit. The "extra" means it comes from a single source. Extra virgin olive oil is beneficial for high blood pressure because it contains more vitamin E than virgin, pure or extra light varieties.

Dilution: Can be used at 100% or 25-50% dilution with another carrier oil blend.

SHEA BUTTER

Shea Butter is a thick, lustrous butter (not a carrier oil) with excellent therapeutic properties. It contains powerful anti-inflammatory properties known to reduce swelling and pain. Shea butter leaves the skin feeling smooth and healthy and combats many skin conditions. Shea butter has a very cream-like consistency, so you may want to warm it and blend it with other carrier oils for a thinner or liquid consistency if desired.

Dilution: Can be used at 100% or diluted at 20-25% with another carrier oil for blending purposes.

TIP: Mineral oil and petroleum jelly should never be used as a carrier oil in therapeutic blending. These are derivatives of petroleum products from gasoline and are not of natural botanical origins. It prevents toxins from escaping the body through perspiration and is believed to also prevent the body from adequately absorbing vitamins and utilizing them, including essential oil absorption.

Carrier oils provide the much-needed lubrication, allowing hands to move freely over the skin, and helping with the absorption of essential oils into the body.

9 / ESSENTIAL OIL SAFETY

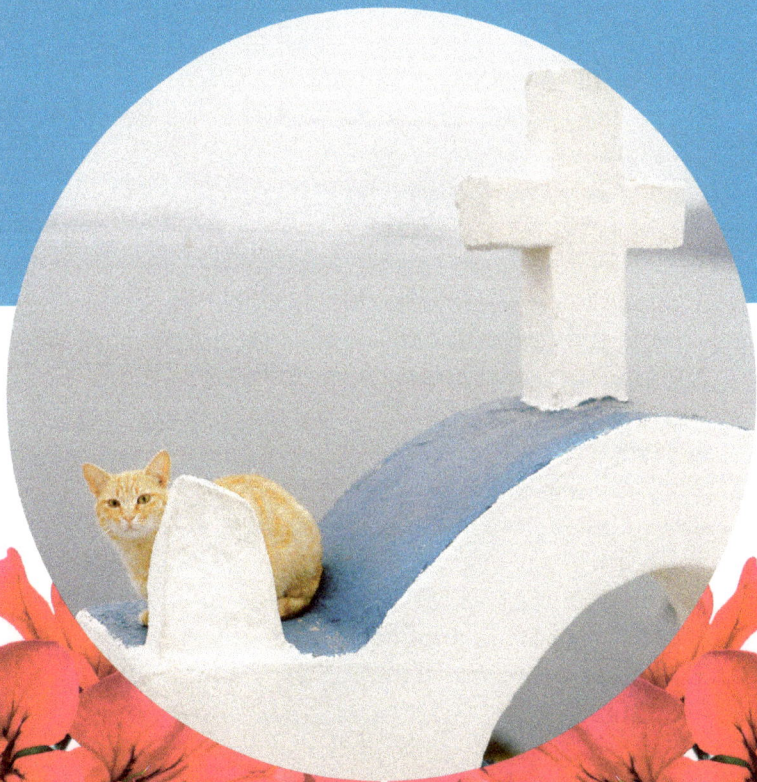

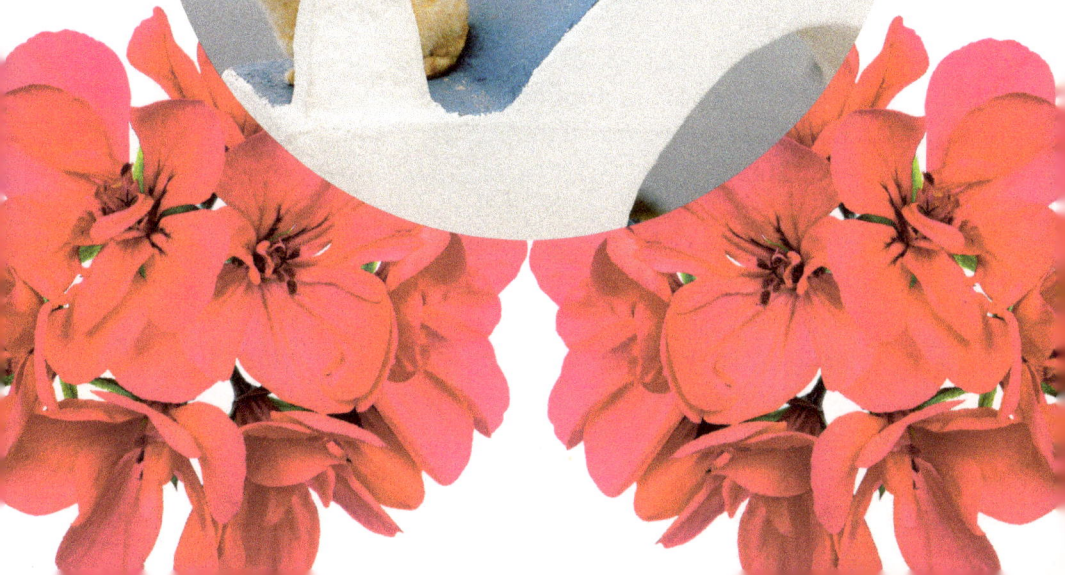

ESSENTIAL OIL SAFETY

Most of the time, essential oils are generally safe for aromatherapy and therapeutic uses. But due to the potency and extreme concentration of the oils, it is recommended to be cautious and exercise safety. Reading the following guidelines will help to avoid all risks that may be associated with essential oils.

- Sunbathing, saunas, or tanning booths can pose threats to the skin and should be avoided after topical application.
- Avoid getting essential oils in the eyes. If essential oils get in the eyes, using a carrier oil such as olive oil (or any other carrier oil) will dilute the essential oil. Use a washcloth to absorb all oil. If severe, seek medical attention at once.
- Due to the strength of essential oils, it is never recommended to use essential oils undiluted on children, and always store essential oils out of reach of children.
- If a large amount of essential oil has been ingested, immediately drink olive oil to induce vomiting. Olive oil will slow the absorption of oil and dilute the essential oil. Do not drink water. This will increase the speed of absorption.
- Most essential oils should be diluted before being used topically. Safety guidelines for some essential oils, Cinnamon and Clove, are known to be irritating for sensitive skin. Stop using oil immediately if there is redness, burning, itching, or irritation. If the skin is irritated, apply olive oil (or any carrier oil) on an area to help reduce absorption. Wipe any remaining oil off the skin with a washcloth. Never use water to dilute oils, as

water only adds to the speed of absorption and can enlarge the affected area.

- If you are pregnant, lactating, suffer from epilepsy, have cancer, liver damage, or another medical condition, use essential oils under the care and supervision of a qualified Aromatherapist or medical practitioner.
- Some essential oils can interact with prescription drugs; check for interaction between the drugs and essential oils (if any) to avoid a conflict with the prescription medications.
- Repeated use of essential oils in the same place can cause irritation or redness of the skin, and it is recommended to use different oils and rotate to prevent this.
- Less is best when ingesting essential oils. Take fewer drops every 4-6 hours versus more at one time.

ESSENTIAL OIL PRECAUTIONS

Essential oils are very potent; some can be harmful in large doses or irritate some people's skin. Various factors are at play to affect anyone that uses essential oils that are directly from age, health concerns, medications, and supplements.

Essential oils always work in conduction with the body, and always paying attention to what certain essential oils affect is highly recommended. For example, some essential oils are known to reduce blood pressure, and those who are using blood thinner medication are at risk of dangerously low levels when using the oils.

Some oils are highly potent; Oregano is one such oil that is not recommended to be used on the skin without dilution for safe use.

ESSENTIAL OILS STORAGE

Essential oils break down over time, often accelerated by heat, light, and air. Following these storage tips can help the essential oils to have prolonged life and maintain their quality for years.

STORAGE TIPS:

- Keep a tight lid on essential oils and keep them out of reach of children.
- Follow and read all labeled cautions and warnings.
- Avoid purchasing essential oils that come with rubber glass dropper tops, as essential oils are very potent and can break down the rubber to a gum which will ruin the essential oil contents.
- Make a note of when the essential oil was opened and how long its shelf-life is.
- Essential oils can remove furniture finish and can cause discoloration. Use care when opening essential oil bottles.
- Keep essential oils stored in a box or a dark place.

Also, it's worth noting to be aware of the quality of essential oils that you purchase. Quality can vary from company to company. In addition, be skeptical of companies claiming their essential oils are pure and undiluted when that claim is false.

Be sure to check for interaction between any prescription medication you are taking and any essential oils you may use to avoid a contraindication.

10 / METHODS OF USE FOR ANXIETY

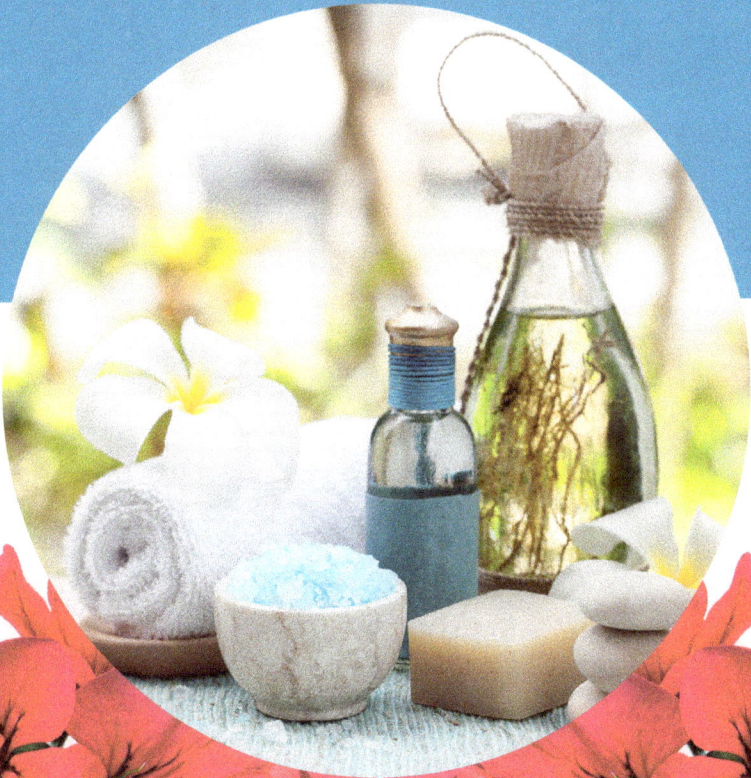

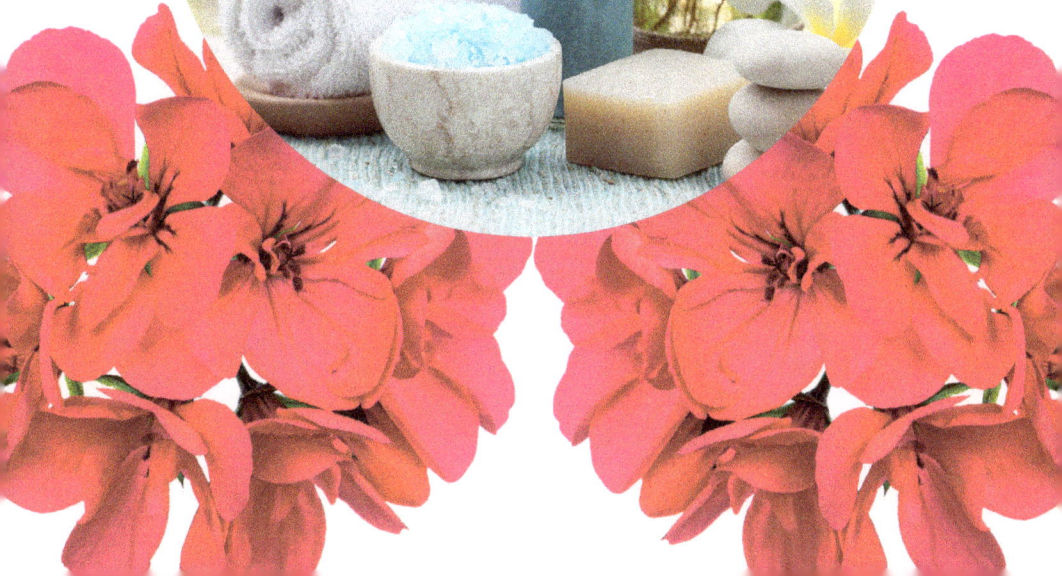

Incorporating essential oils and natural remedies such as aromatherapy and relaxation techniques into your life can be very beneficial for anxiety. When used correctly, most essential oils are safe and free of adverse side effects. However, as with any substance you introduce into your body, it is necessary to use them intelligently.

Most essential oils that have sedative or relaxing qualities may be used to help bring stress relief. If you suffer from chronic stress, you might find additional essential oils to combine in your blend with the oils suggested. For example, you may want to combine Bergamot (Citrus bergamia) or Sweet Orange (Citrus sinensis) in a depression-related stress relief blend since these essential oils uplift the emotional system while relaxing the body.

HERE ARE SOME FACTORS TO CONSIDER:

Dosage – Dose is the most significant factor in essential oil usage. Some essential oils used in the wrong doses, such as in too high of a concentration, have been found (in animal and laboratory studies) to cause adverse effects on the body. Some essential oils can damage the skin, liver, and other organs if misused.

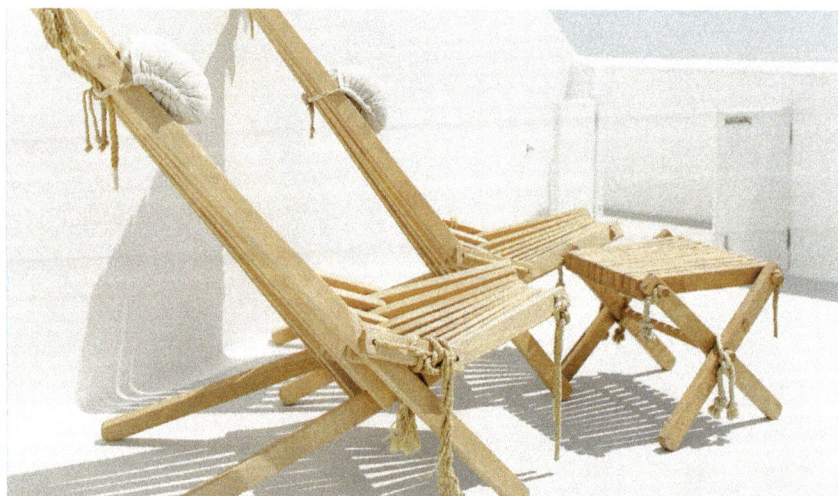

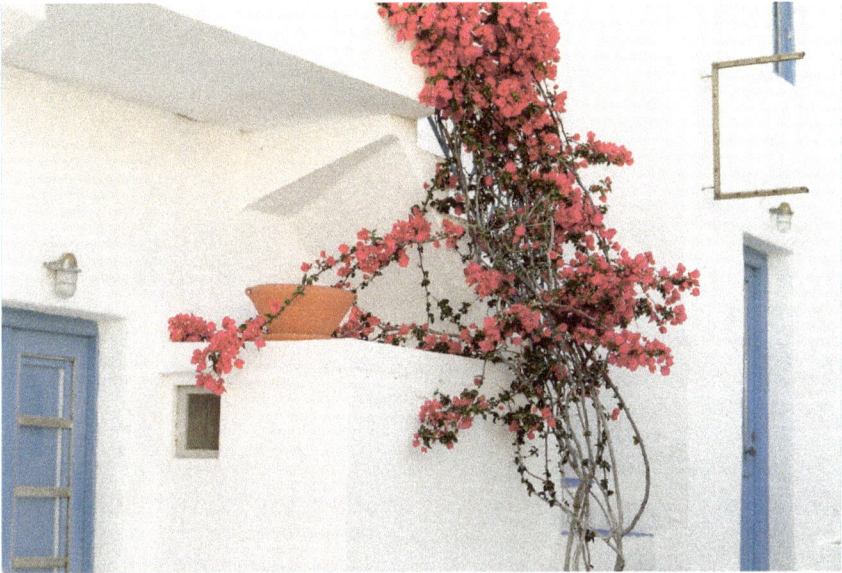

Quality – The purity of the essential oil is important. Even when oil is labeled as pure, it may be adulterated with added synthetic chemicals or similar smelling, cheaper essential oils or vegetable oil. Make sure your oils are of therapeutic quality.

Application – An essential oil that is safe when applied in one way may not be safe when used in another way. Some oils are considered safe if inhaled and yet may be irritating if applied to the skin in concentration. For instance, citrus oils such as Bergamot and Lemon can cause phototoxicity (severe burn to the skin) if a person is exposed to the sun after topical application. However, this would not result from inhalation.

Lifestyle – Chronic stress is a debilitating health condition. It is important to combine your use of essential oils with diet and lifestyle changes to achieve success with your natural remedy.

Drug Interaction – If you're currently under a doctor's care, talk to your doctor before starting any treatment program with essential oils. You will want to ensure that your oils will not interfere with the prescribed medications.

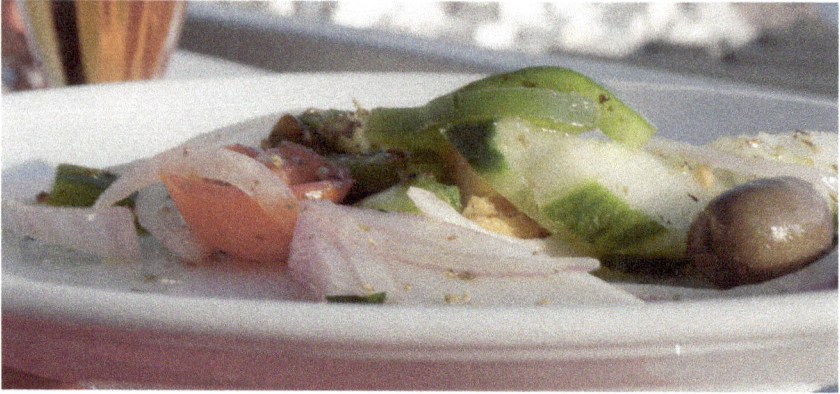

Another option is to find a naturopath to talk to that looks at your health as a whole instead of treating symptoms of individual conditions. As you study and research therapeutic quality essential oils, you will find these are a great way to complement your whole-body care instead of taking a handful of pills daily for multiple medical issues.

The suggestions for essential oils in this book are for you to use as complementary care to the healthcare plan you already have. You may need to change your diet and other lifestyle modifications for all things to work together. If you do not achieve satisfactory results in improving stress, please seek professional medical help.

Several options are available for treating stress in both allopathic and alternative medicine. Many people today can improve their stress-related symptoms with the help of therapeutic quality essential oils along with vigilance and commitment to a healthy diet and lifestyle.

Various mechanisms can be used to deliver essential oils to target sites in the body. Typical routes of administration include inhalation, topical, and ingestion. Regardless of which route of administration is used, the essential oils have to travel to the site of action with either the help of blood, nerves, or oxygen (when the inhalation route is used). Combining these three approaches will ensure success.

11 / AROMATIC USE

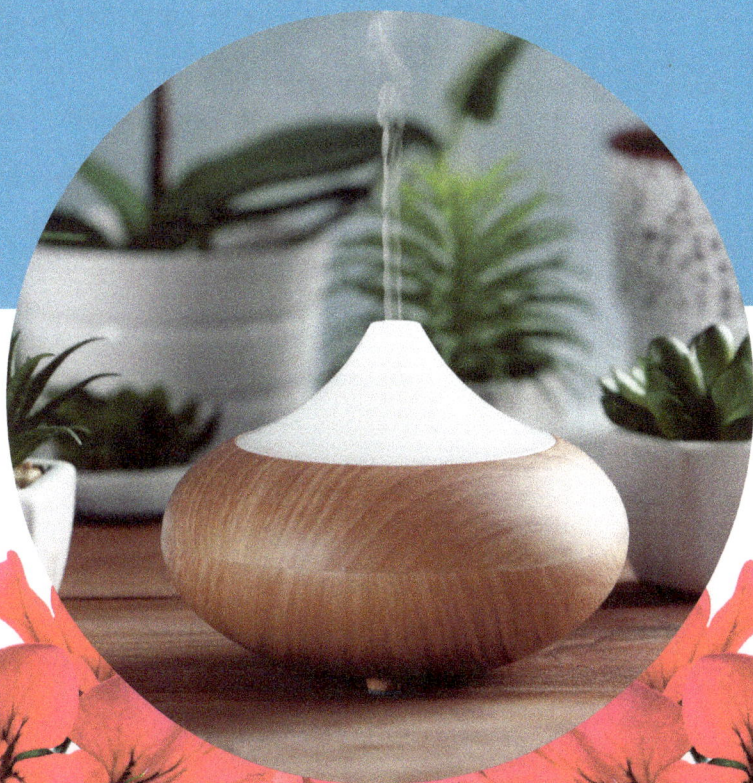

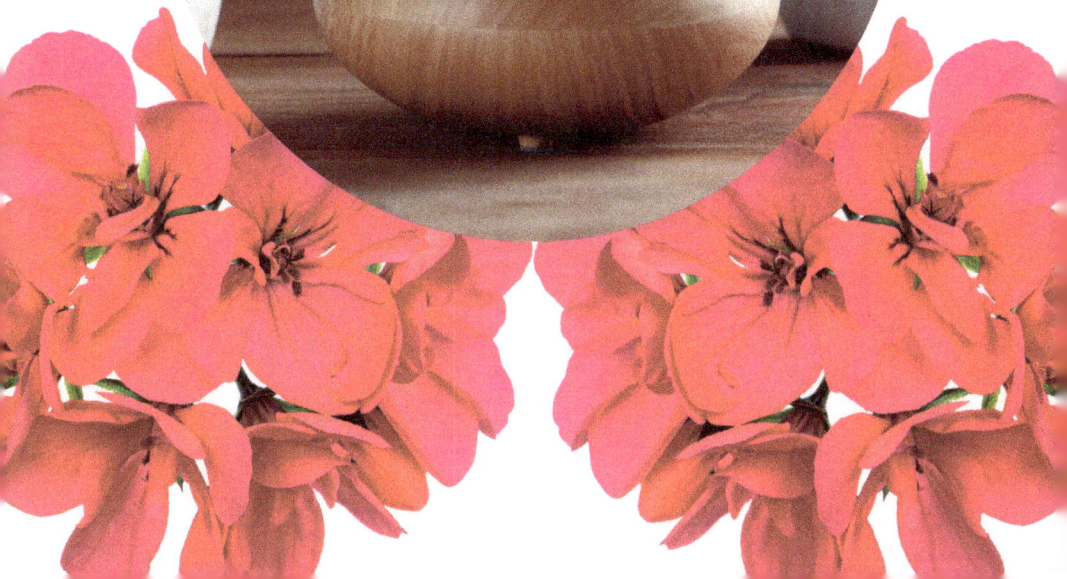

Inhalation is one of the most natural methods of use and is considered the most direct pathway for an aromatic blend or essence. When inhaled, fragrant vapors enter the lungs and are instantly released into the bloodstream for delivery to every cell in the body. Scientific research shows that essential oils can remain in a person's bloodstream for up to 4-6 hours, depending on the essential oil.

Essential oils that are adequately diffused are known to improve mental clarity, enhance or calm emotions, and increase feelings of well-being. If a diffuser is not available, making a room spray, personal inhaler, or placing a few drops on a tissue to inhale will suffice. All are very effective ways to benefit from the therapeutic properties of essential oils. For inhalation, use intermittent exposure (less than 15 minutes in an hour).

Inhalation of certain essential oil vapors triggers the olfactory bulb, which immediately sends a neurochemical signal to neuro-receptors. For example, smelling Lavender essential oil .triggers the release of serotonin from the raphe nucleus in the brain and produces a calmative effect. Essential oils can easily be absorbed via inhalation and enter the bloodstream to deliver healing constituents throughout the body. Inhalation presents the least amount of risk for most individuals.

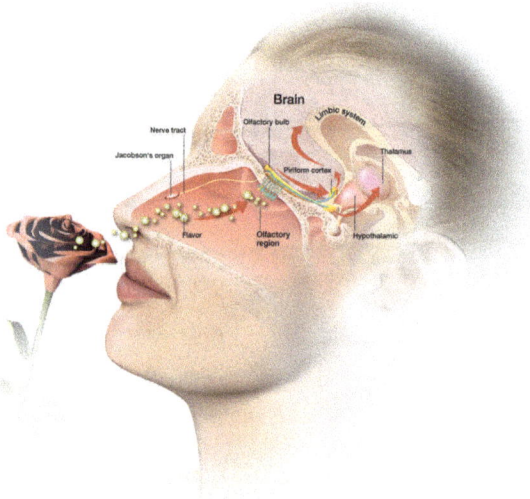

Some of the ways to use essential oils for anxiety include the following:

- **Diffuser** – Try adding essential oil or a blend of choice to a diffuser. Use a nebulizer to diffuse your selection of oils for an hour three times a day. You may want to use one specific essential oil (with no carrier oil added). Or you may blend a combination of essential oils. Place 10-12 essential oil into a diffuser in the bedroom and run for 15 minutes before work or bed.
- **Cup Hands** – Place 2-3 drops of your chosen essential oil in your hand and rub your palms together. Cup hands over your nose and inhale deeply.
- **Personal Inhaler** – Add 1-2 drops of essential oil to a tissue and carry it with you to smell throughout the day, or add several drops of pure essential oil to a pocket diffuser and use it 2-3 times daily.
- **Room Spray** – Spritz your home office, living room, pillow, and bedsheets with a relaxing fragrance.
- **Smelling Salts** – In a small tub or 10 ml (1/3 oz.) glass bottle, add 30 drops of the essential oil blend and fill the remainder with either fine or coarse sea salt. Waft the bottle under your nose while inhaling deeply whenever you need to calm your mind.
- **Shower Steamers** – Make these ahead and drop them in a hot shower or bath to relax. You can also add a few drops of a relaxing essential oil to Epsom salts for a nice bedtime bath!
- **Cotton Ball** – Add a few drops to a tissue or cotton ball and tuck it inside your pillowcase. Add a drop of Roman Chamomile essential oil or Lavender essential oil to a tissue or cotton ball and place that near your pillow at bedtime. Roman Chamomile essential oil is considered a natural sedative. Another essential oil that possesses sedating properties is Clary Sage essential oil.
- **Bottle** – Open the bottle and take a sniff several times when you need quick anxiety relief.
- **Humidifier / Vaporizer** – Place ten drops of essential oil undiluted into the unit for a humidifier or vaporizer.

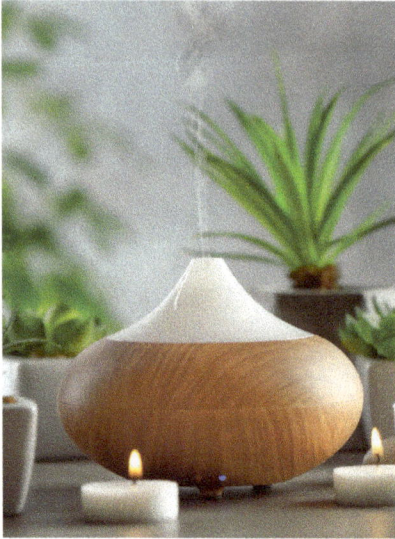

DIFFUSER BLENDS

Pleasant, relaxing aromas used in a diffuser are one of the most effective ways to lessen anxiety. The diffuser transforms the oil into a fine mist of oil droplets which disperse the scent throughout the air. This enables you to enjoy its pleasing aroma for an extended time, making it the most convenient way to use essential oils for anxiety.

There are plenty of essential oil diffusers to choose from. Before buying one, evaluate your needs to determine which model will serve you best. Be sure the diffuser doesn't heat the oil as this may change its molecular structure, rendering it less potent and effective (glass nebulizer, waterless is best).

If you have other health conditions, you may want to consult with a certified aromatherapist before using essential oils aromatically. Essential oils can be highly potent, and adverse reactions may occur.

BLENDING ESSENTIAL OILS

Combining several essential oils in one diffuser is one way to enjoy the benefits of essential oil diffusion. Blending your diffuser blend creates a new aroma that

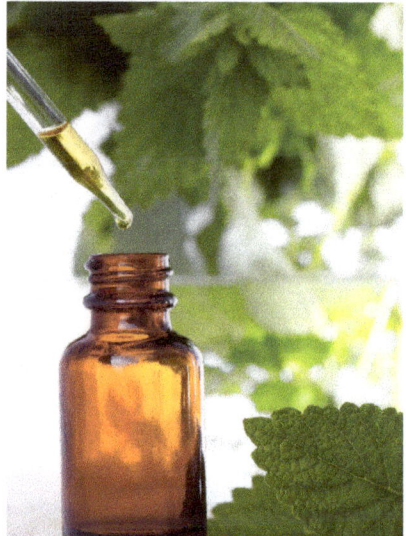

is unique and different. The number of combinations you can make are limitless, but it might be challenging to know which oils pair well with others and which don't. For best results, follow the instructions below to learn how to make essential oil blends at home.

TIPS FOR MAKING A GOOD DIFFUSER BLEND

1. Determine the desired effect you want from the diffuser blend. The oil you use will determine the feeling you want to experience, such as relaxing, calming, or invigorating.

   Are you trying to create a calming environment? Once you determine the desired outcome, choosing oils complementing one another will be easier.

2. Choose a group of oils with similar properties to help you achieve your desired effect. If you want a relaxing diffuser blend, choose oils known for calmness and serenity, like Lavender. Choose oils with stimulating properties like Peppermint or Lemon if you want an energizing effect.

3. Once you have decided on the oils you want to use, you can begin pairing them together.

Pairing Different Oils: When you want to add variety to your essential oil blends, you can pair oils from different categories together for various new aromas. As you blend oils from different categories, you can end up with a unique blend that showcases the best attributes of each oil.

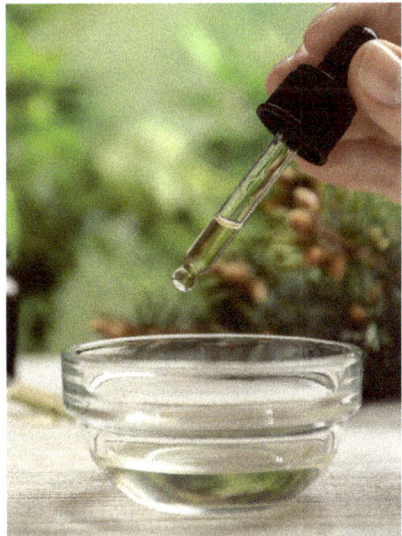

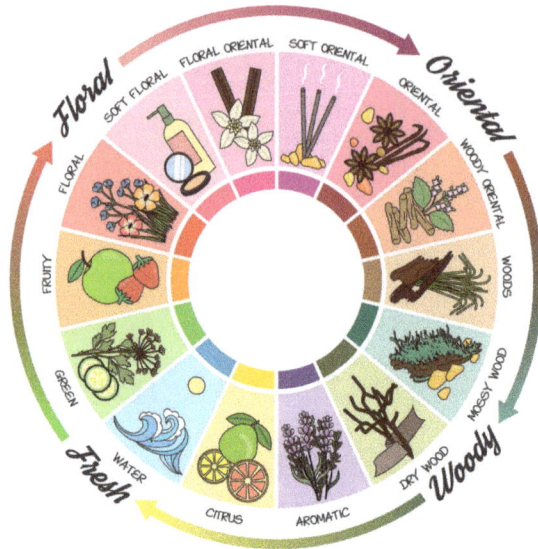

PAIRING OILS FROM DIFFERENT CATEGORIES:

- ♦ Floral oils blend well with spicy, woody, and citrus oils
- ♦ Spicy oils blend well with citrus, woody, and floral oils
- ♦ Citrus oils blend well with woody, floral, spicy, and mint oils
- ♦ Herbaceous essential oils blend well with mint and woody oils
- ♦ Mint essential oils blend well with woody, earthy, herbaceous, and citrus oils

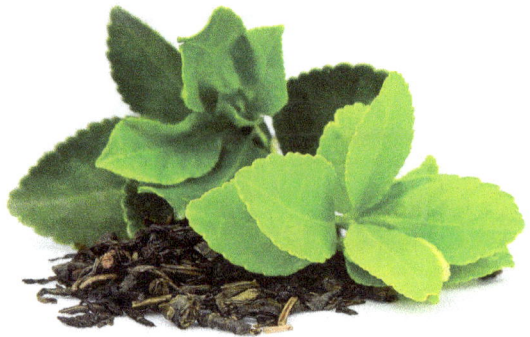

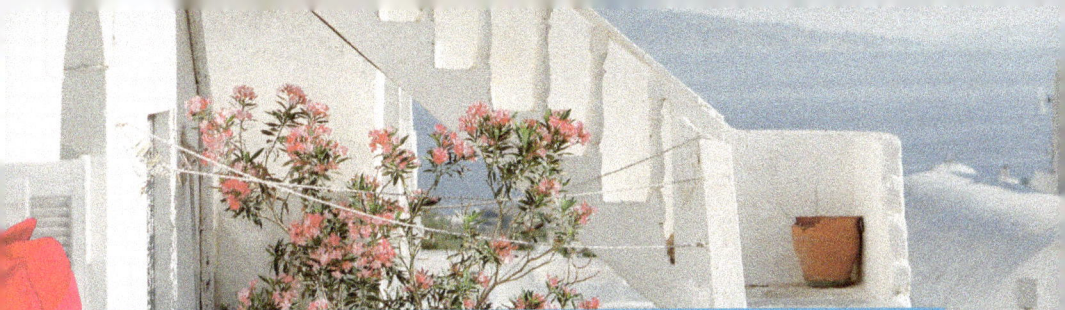

BLEND BY EFFECT

When creating a diffuser or inhaler blend, combine essential oils for the same effect. For example, to create a relaxing blend, you might try blending Lemon (top), Marjoram (middle), and Jasmine (base). These all fall within the same category, Relaxing, so you know they will pair well together.

PEACEFUL

Lavender, Sandalwood, Roman Chamomile, Ylang Ylang, Rose, Lemon Verbena, Orange, Patchouli, Blue Tansy, Bergamot, Clary Sage, Niaouli, Frankincense, Geranium, Cedarwood, Benzoin, Jasmine, Tangerine, Neroli, and Marjoram

RELAXING

Lavender, Sandalwood, Roman Chamomile, Ylang Ylang, Tangerine, Rose, Lemon Verbena, Patchouli, Bergamot, Clary Sage, Geranium, Benzoin, Jasmine, Neroli, Marjoram, Melissa, Petitgrain, Citronella, and Yarrow

ENERGIZING

Rosemary, Peppermint, Lemon, Lime, Balsam Pine, Orange, Thyme, Jasmine, Myrrh, Cardamom, Bergamot, Cypress, Marjoram, and Eucalyptus

STIMULATING & INVIGORATING

Bergamot, Orange, Rosemary, Lemon Verbena, Spearmint, Sage, Pine, Cypress, Ginger, Grapefruit, Clary Sage, Lemon, Basil, Frankincense, Patchouli, Black Pepper, Wintergreen, and Sandalwood

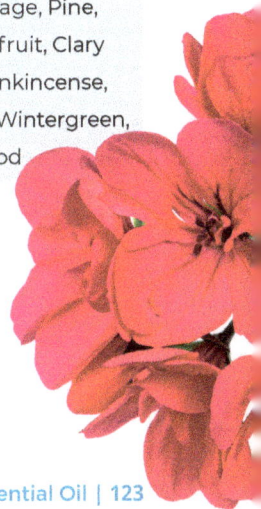

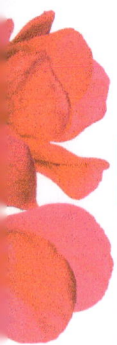

MENTAL CLARITY

Frankincense, Peppermint, Rosemary, Grapefruit, Lemon, Lemongrass, Roman Chamomile, Cinnamon, Orange, Bergamot, Black Pepper, Basil, Eucalyptus, Vetiver, and Ylang Ylang

FOCUS & CONCENTRATION

Lemon, Fennel, Thyme, Grapefruit, Bergamot, Basil, Cypress, Cinnamon, Peppermint, Cedarwood, Lemongrass, Eucalyptus, and Nutmeg

ROMANTIC & EXOTIC

Ylang Ylang, Rose, Jasmine, Cassia, Cinnamon, Sandalwood, Orange, Vanilla, Bergamot, Neroli, and Patchouli

JOYFUL & HAPPY

Orange, Rose, Jasmine, Ginger, Clove, Cinnamon, Sandalwood, Frankincense, Lemon, Bergamot, Lime, Grapefruit, and Petitgrain

POSITIVE & CONFIDENT

Cypress, Fennel, Ginger, Grapefruit, Jasmine, Orange, Basil, Lemon, Myrrh, Patchouli, Geranium, Frankincense, and Pine

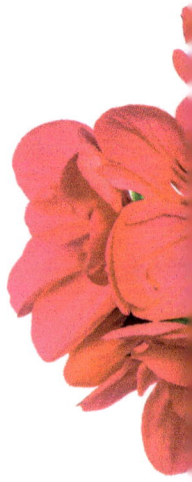

DIFFUSER BLEND RECIPES

CHILL ZONE

- 4 drops Lavender essential oil
- 4 drops Frankincense essential oil
- 1 drop Bergamot essential oil
- 1 drop Ylang Ylang essential oil

STRESS RELIEF

- 3 drops Lemon essential oil
- 2 drops Grapefruit essential oil
- 1 drop Spearmint essential oil

CRUSHING IT

- 2 drops Lemon essential oil
- 3 drops Lavender essential oil
- 3 drops Geranium essential oil

FREE THE MIND

- 3 drops Lavender essential oil
- 3 drops Orange essential oil
- 2 drops Geranium essential oil

BREATHE & RELAX

- 3 drops Lavender essential oil
- 3 drops Bergamot essential oil
- 2 drops Ylang Ylang essential oil

WINDING DOWN

- 4 drops Frankincense essential oil
- 3 drops Clary Sage essential oil
- 3 drops Litsea essential oil

INNER PEACE

- 4 drops Grapefruit essential oil
- 3 drops Frankincense essential oil
- 3 drops Patchouli essential oil

LOVING THYSELF

- 3 drops Clary Sage essential oil
- 2 drops Geranium essential oil
- 2 drops Petitgrain essential oil

GOING WITH THE FLOW

- 3 drops Cypress essential oil
- 2 drops Lemongrass essential oil
- 2 drops Orange essential oil

OCEAN WAVES

- 3 drops Lavender essential oil
- 3 drops Lime essential oil
- 1 drop Spearmint essential oil

STAY ON TRACK

- 3 drops Frankincense essential oil
- 3 drops Bergamot essential oil
- 2 drops Sandalwood essential oil

INHALE & EXHALE

- 2 drops Juniper Berry essential oil
- 2 drops Grapefruit essential oil
- 1 drop Douglas Fir essential oil

PERSONAL INHALERS

Essential oil inhalers are an excellent way to enjoy the perks of essential oils even when you're not at home or unable to use a diffuser. They're portable, practical, and discreet. Plastic inhalers are typically made of four parts: a cover, a wick, a wick enclosure, and a cap. Aluminum inhalers are generally made of a glass vial, a wick, an aluminum screw-on top with air holes, an outer aluminum enclosure, and an aluminum cap.

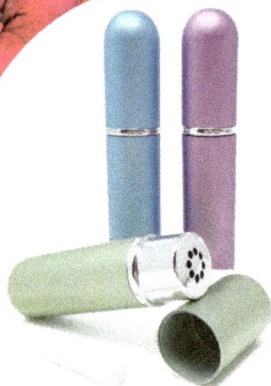

What You Will Need:

Inhaler apparatus
Label
Essential oils for the blend you choose (up to 15 drops)
Tiny bowl
Pipette
Tweezers

What To Do:

1. Mix the essential oils for your chosen blend in a tiny bowl.
2. Place the wick in the bowl.
3. Using your tweezers, rotate the wick around to absorb the essential oil blend completely.
4. Once the wick is saturated with the oil, use the tweezers to pick it up and place it in the wick enclosure (the part with a hole at the top).
5. Secure the end cap or butt onto the wick enclosure.
6. Screw the outer cover onto the wick enclosure.
7. Label your inhaler.
8. Keep the lid/cover on the inhaler when you are not using it.

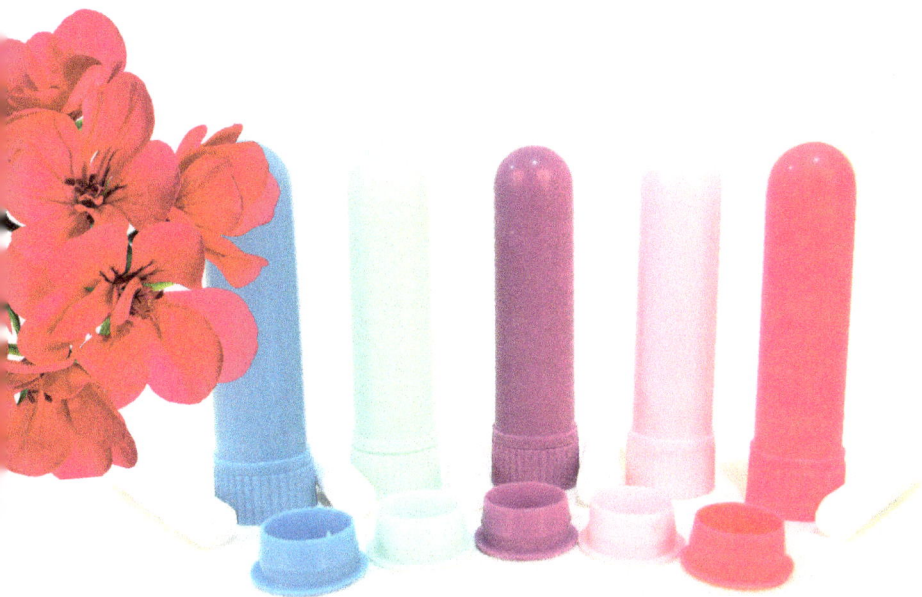

HOW TO USE YOUR ESSENTIAL OIL INHALER:

- Remove the cap from your essential oil inhaler.
- Raise it to one nostril, ensuring that the tip of the inhaler does not come into direct contact with your nose (or other skin).
- Inhale as deeply as is comfortable.
- Repeat with the other nostril.
- Close the cap.
- If you experience any adverse reactions, discontinue using your inhaler immediately.

Check the safety information to ensure the oil is appropriate for personal use. The essential oil blends suggested in this book are for healthy adults with no serious underlying medical issues. For children, cut the number of drops in half. Inhaler blends are not recommended for children under six.

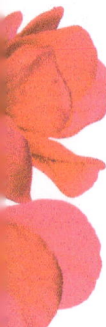

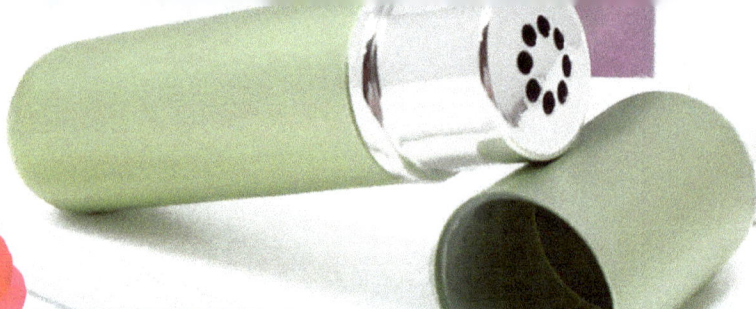

PERSONAL INHALER BLENDS

CHILLING

- 5 drops Sweet Orange essential oil
- 5 drops Cedarwood essential oil
- 1 drop Ylang Ylang essential oil
- 1 drop Patchouli essential oil

SLEEP LIKE BABY

- 5 drops Clary Sage essential oil
- 2 drops Lavender essential oil
- 5 drops Bergamot essential oil

SWEET SURRENDER

- 6 drops Lavender essential oil
- 4 drops Cypress essential oil
- 4 drops Marjoram essential oil
- 2 drops Wintergreen essential oil

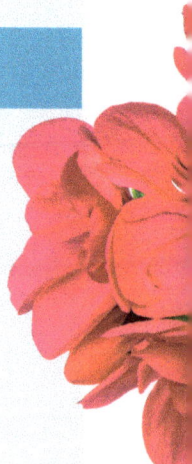

FEELING GROUNDED

- 6 drops Lavender essential oil
- 4 drops Myrrh essential oil
- 4 drops Roman Chamomile essential oil

CITRUSY BOOST

- 5 drops Bergamot essential oil
- 5 drops Neroli essential oil
- 5 drops Sandalwood essential oil

ANXIETY BE GONE

- 4 drops Lavender essential oil
- 4 drops Clary Sage essential oil
- 2 drops Frankincense essential oil

LIFTING YOU UP

- 5 drops Bergamot essential oil
- 3 drops Clary Sage essential oil
- 2 drops Ylang Ylang essential oil

CALM DOWN

- 6 drops Mandarin essential oil
- 2 drops Ylang Ylang essential oil
- 2 drops Patchouli essential oil

GOOD MORNING

- 5 drops Grapefruit essential oil
- 5 drops Frankincense essential oil
- 5 drops Patchouli essential oil

DRIFT AWAY

- 5 drops Lavender essential oil
- 4 drops Cypress essential oil
- 4 drops Marjoram essential oil
- 2 drops Wintergreen essential oil

ROOM SPRAY

A room spray is a type of diffusion that quickly releases a concentrated amount of oil into the air. You will use approximately 30-40 drops of essential oil in hydrosol, mineral water, or vodka. Use as needed to create a special atmosphere.

To ensure the essential oils disperse throughout the hydrosol or another water-based carrier (and stay mixed), you will need to add a product called Solubol, an all-natural dispersant.

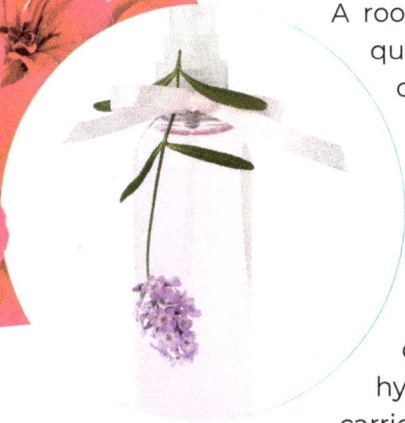

What You Will Need:

18 - 24 drops Top Note Essential Oil
12 - 16 drops Middle Note Essential Oil
6 - 8 drops Base Note Essential oil
2 oz (60 ml) Glass Spray Bottle
1/2 teaspoon Solubol or Aloe Vera Gel
Glass Bowl
Stir Rod
Funnel
2 oz Hydrosol, Floral Water, or Distilled Water

What To Do:

1. Remove the spray nozzle from the spray bottle—you will add your carrier and oils right into the spray bottle.
2. Choose three essential oils. Add the number of drops for each note. Check the scent when adding drops to make sure you are happy with the scent.
3. Replace the nozzle and cap and shake.
4. Create a nice label for your room spray.

> *When creating a relaxing diffuser blend, combine essential oils for the same effect, such as peaceful or relaxing.*

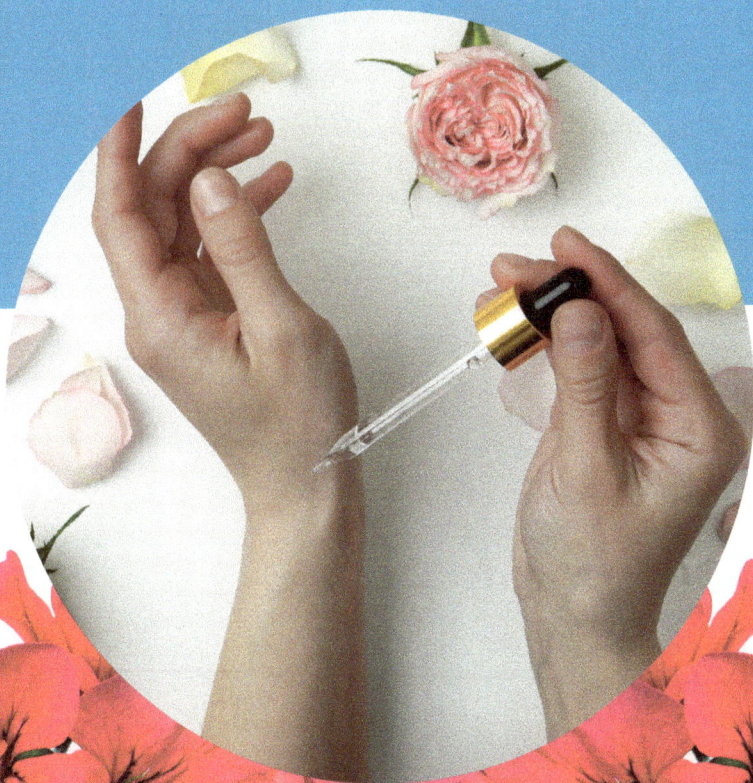

12 / TOPICAL USE

Topical use is applying the essential oils directly to the skin's surface; always use a carrier for topical use. Ways to use essential oils topically include:

- ◆ Roller Bottle
- ◆ Lotion
- ◆ Massage Oil
- ◆ Bath Salts

You can apply the essential oil(s) of choice to the back of the neck, feet, legs, etc., mixed with a lotion or carrier oil. Try combining a couple of oils to create a synergistic blend for multiple health benefits.

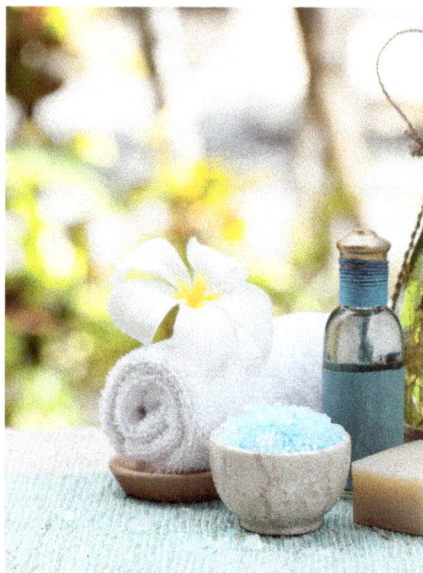

When using an essential oil topically, dilute it with a carrier oil. Essential oils are potent and direct application, or "neat," may cause irritation to the skin. Also, combining essential oils with a carrier base oil such as almond or coconut oil can add additional benefits to your treatment.

Topical use is one of the easiest and most effective ways to use essential oils. For example, massage stimulates blood circulation while reducing muscular tension, aches and pain, and inflammation. Also, it significantly reduces anxiousness and can offer comfort and peace of mind, allowing you to sleep. Caution should be exercised when using topical aromatherapy preparations around drug injection sites or areas of the body where transdermal medications are in use (i.e., estrogen or nicotine patches, etc.).

The absorption of certain essential oil chemical compounds has been confirmed through analysis of blood concentrations, with maximum levels attained in as little as 10 minutes.

- **Roll-On** – Use a rollerball applicator to apply the oil blend where needed. Reapply several times a day as needed.
- **Rub On** – Rub 1-2 drops of essential oil directly "neat" on the joint or affected area. Or rub an essential oil or essential oil blend on the bottom of your feet each evening before bed.
- **Massage** – Massage an essential oil blend (with a carrier oil) over the body for several minutes. Reapply as desired. Apply to the back of the neck, joints, and feet. Applying essential oils topically can be beneficial since they will permeate your skin due to their transdermal properties. Massage and therapeutic baths will be your best methods of treatment. They stimulate circulation, help eliminate toxins, and absorb the minerals needed to function correctly. A variety of techniques used in massage therapy can incorporate the use of essential oils. Add 6-9 drops of essential oil to a tablespoon of your favorite carrier oil to massage into the body.
- **Bath** – Sea salt baths are great for relaxation because they stimulate circulation. For a full bath, mix 8-10 drops of essential oil into two ounces of sea salts or a cup of milk, then pour into a running bath. Agitate water in a figure-eight motion to make sure the oil is mixed well, preventing irritation to mucous membranes. Another method is to add essential oils after the bath has been drawn. Mix essential oils into a palm full of liquid soap, shampoo, or a tablespoon of Jojoba oil and swish around to dissolve in the tub. Soak for 15-20 minutes. Adding salts to the bath helps relax muscles which can help you to relax.
- **Shower** – While showering, add a drop or two of essential oil to a washcloth with liquid soap or body wash and rub it on the body.

- **Lotion** – Blending essential oils in an unscented, natural lotion/cream base allows you to benefit from the therapeutic qualities of the essential oil, giving you a non-oily way to apply essential oils. This is especially useful for someone with a skin condition that does not do well with oils. The dilution rate for using essential oils in a lotion base is no more than 2%. For adults, use 20 drops of essential oil to four ounces of lotion. For children and the elderly, use ten drops of essential oil to four ounces of lotion.
- **Body Oil** – Mix 30 drops of essential oil per ounce of cold-pressed carrier oil, such as coconut oil. Choose an all-purpose oil that relieves anxiousness, tension, and headaches and smells terrific.

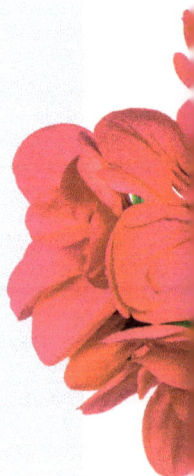

MASSAGE OIL

Essential oils have been used for many years to enhance relaxation during a massage. An essential oil with a calming, relaxing property as part of a relaxing massage is a great way to relieve anxiety.

To apply, warm a few drops of essential oil with a teaspoon of your favorite carrier oil in your hand, rub between the palms, and then massage the oil into the temples or neck muscles. Massaging these two areas with essential oils is an effective way to calm and relax you.

This can also be applied to the shoulders, arms, back, legs, or feet to help relax these areas. Diluting essential oils with carrier oil will help the oils be absorbed into the skin and linger after the massage. Please make sure the essential oil you choose is safe for topical use. Some oils are potent and irritate the skin if not recommended for topical use.

As a rule of thumb: Use two to three drops of essential oil per teaspoon of carrier oil (follow individual recipes when available). A full-body massage takes about one to two ounces of carrier oil. Any natural carrier oil (except mineral oil) is okay to use when preparing a massage blend.

When Choosing Your Carrier Oil:

- **Odor:** A few carrier oils have a distinct smell. When added to an essential oil, it may alter the aroma.
- **Absorption:** Your skin can absorb some carrier oils better than others.
- **Skin Type:** Depending on your skin type, some oils may irritate or worsen a skin condition, such as acne.
- **Shelf Life:** Some carrier oils can be stored longer than others without going rancid.

An essential oil with a calming, relaxing property as part of a soothing massage is a great way to relieve anxiety.

13 / ORAL USE

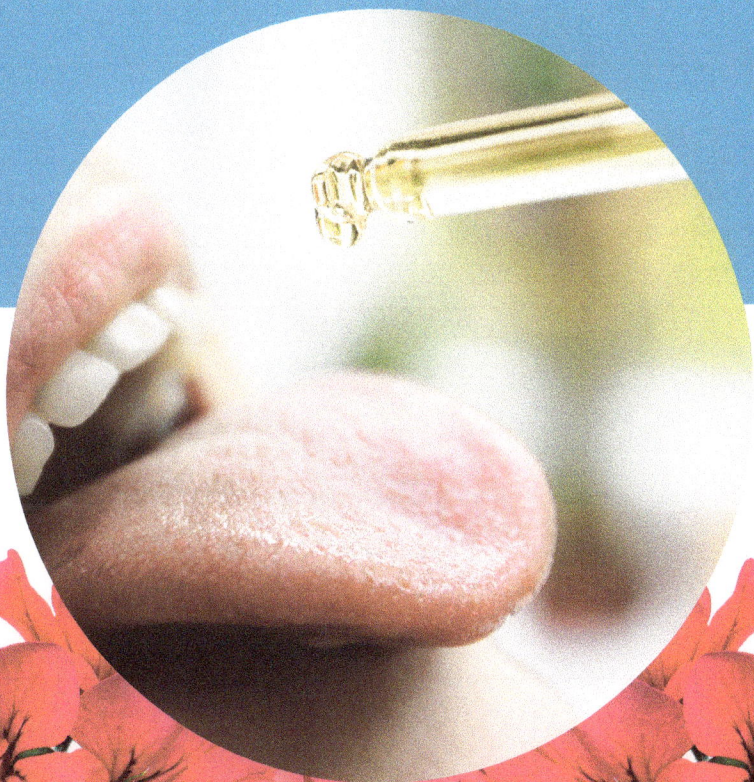
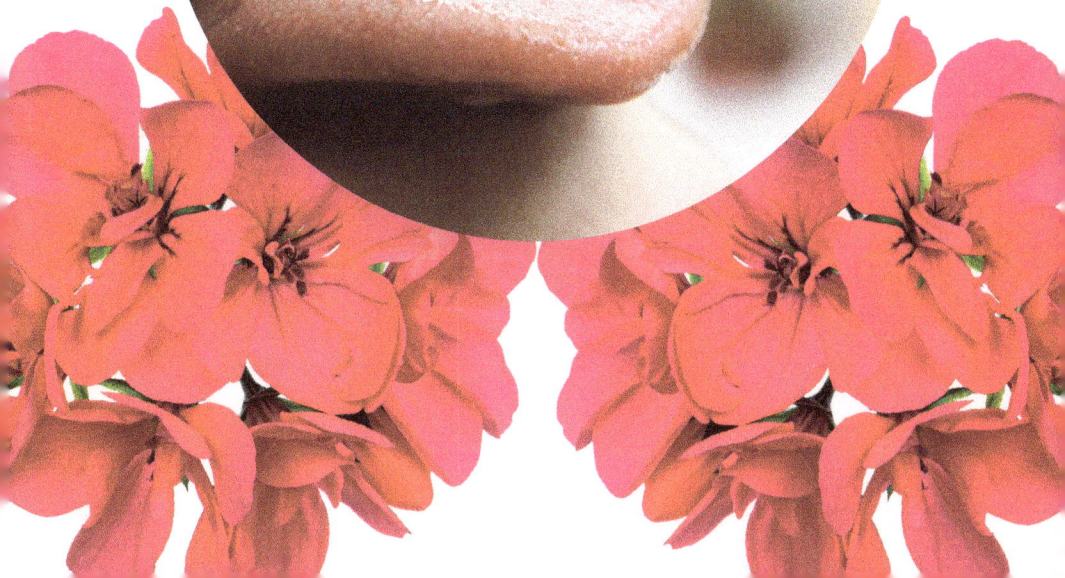

Certain essential oils can be taken internally for relaxation. Please check the label carefully to ensure the essential oil you choose is safe for ingestion. Not all essential oils are safe for taking orally.

If you are considering ingesting essential oils, you will want to treat them like powerful medicines because that is what they are. Taking an oil orally is nearly ten times stronger than when applied topically, so starting with a tiny amount and increasing gradually is wise. While many essential oils are generally considered safe (GRAS) when used internally, some are not. Be sure to research and find out if there are any precautions or contradictions. Also, you will want to be aware of proper dosage protocols. The internal dose and frequency of use will vary based on age, weight, and health condition.

According to one essential oil company, the recommended internal dose of essential oils is 1–5 drops, depending on the oil or blend. Taking more than that is not advantageous; in fact, it can be harmful. It is better to take a smaller dose, which can be repeated every 4–6 hours as needed. A low daily dose is recommended for extended internal use.

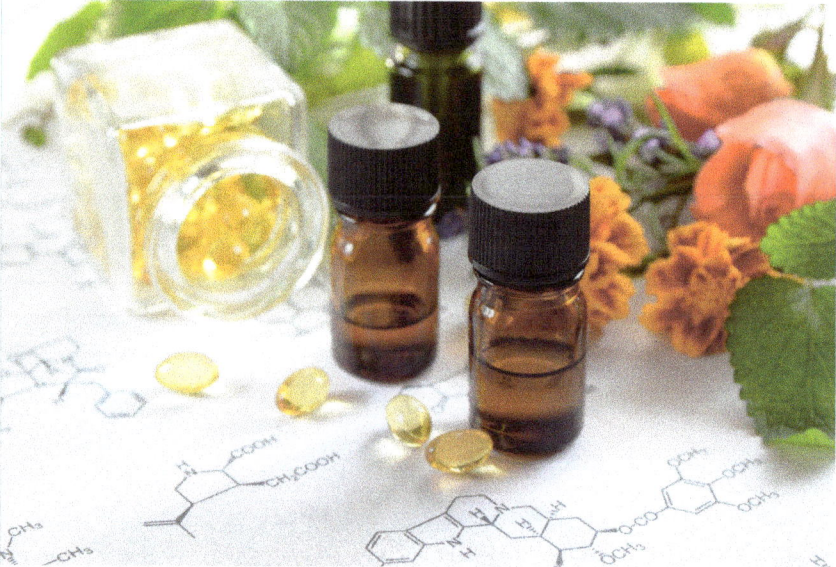

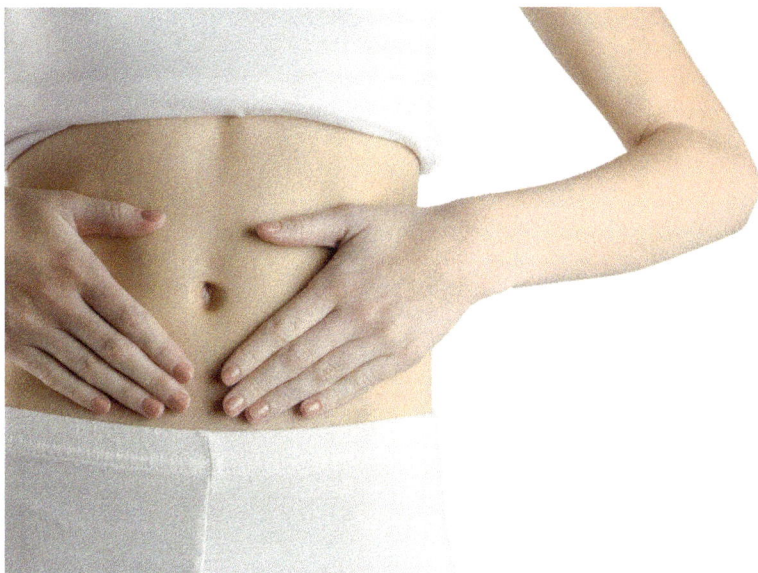

Ingestion of essential oils is not always the most efficient method for absorption into the bloodstream. Due to the first-pass hepatic metabolism, the chemical constituents absorbed into systemic circulation via the digestive tract may lose some active principal compounds.

There are several methods for taking essential oils. In this book, internal use will comprise consuming essential oils by mouth in a vegetable capsule, adding oil to honey, or on a sugar cube. Another method is taking one drop of essential oil by mouth (not in a capsule) to be absorbed through the cheeks, tongue, or throat lining.

Essential oils are highly concentrated and potent—treat like any other highly concentrated pharmaceutical.

When using essential oils internally, a dose ranges from one to three drops, once to twice daily (for a healthy adult). Using the appropriate amount of essential oil in a vegetable capsule that has been adequately diluted can be maximally absorbed by the gut for the whole-body effect. But like medicines, essential oil

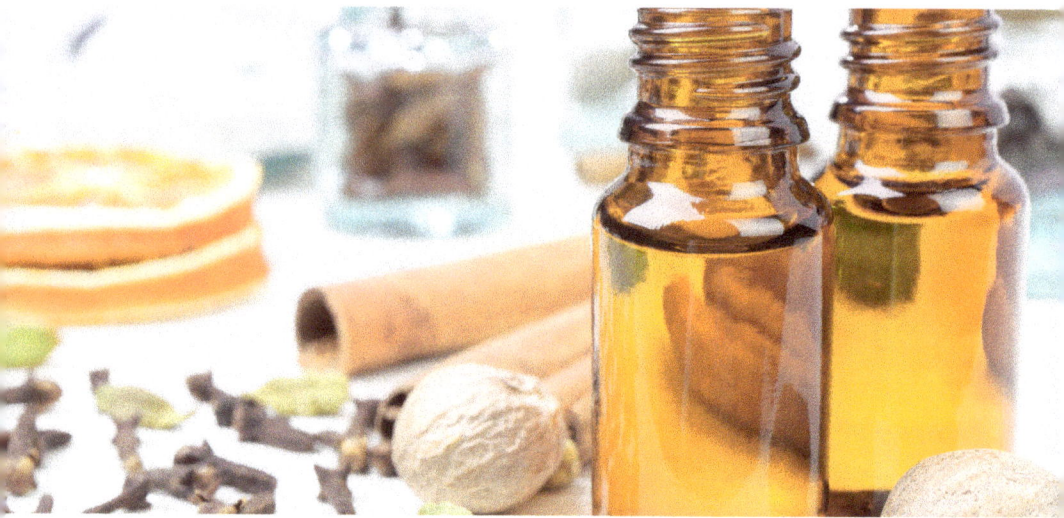

ingestion carries the potential for side effects, mild to severe, including seizures and poisoning.

When using essential oils internally, it is recommended to seek the advice of a certified medical practitioner who is also trained in aromatherapy or a Clinical Certified Aromatherapist who is also trained in internal ingestion for the best protocol. Please store your oils in a safe place away from children.

WAYS TO USE ESSENTIAL OILS ORALLY

Capsules – Add one or two drops of essential oil to a "00" gelatin capsule filled with a carrier oil such as olive or fractionated co-conut oil to buffer the essential oil. Take orally as you would with traditional supplements. A single oil or essential oil blend may be used in this way. For example, a capsule is filled with 20% essential oil diluted with 80% vegetable oil. Each "00" capsule holds approximately 0.7-.91ml or 14 drops, and "0" capsules hold ten drops of oil. Enteric-coated gelatin capsules are recommended since they do not release the essential oil until they reach the small intestine.

Juice or Water – Add one or two drops of essential oil to a small glass of juice. Stir to blend well, as oil will tend to float on the surface. Solubol can be added as a dispersant to distribute the oils.

Tea – Add one or two drops of essential oil to a teaspoon of honey and stir into a cup of tea or warm water. Be sure not to overheat the water, as oils will evaporate. Sip slowly.

Swishing – Add several drops of essential oil to a cup of water and swish around the mouth before swallowing.

Sugar Cube – Use a dropper to add one or two drops of essential oil to a sugar cube. It can be taken directly or added to a drink.

Honey – Essential oils can be blended with honey water. Mix 1-2 drops of essential oil into one teaspoon of honey, add to warm water, and drink. Or add 1-2 drops of essential oil or oil blend to a tablespoon of honey, stir with a toothpick, and take orally.

The recommended oral dosage with essential oils for adults is 1-3 drops, two to three times a day. The maximum daily dose is 12 drops. Some professionals recommend using essential oils two weeks out of the month or taking one drop three times a day for an extended period.

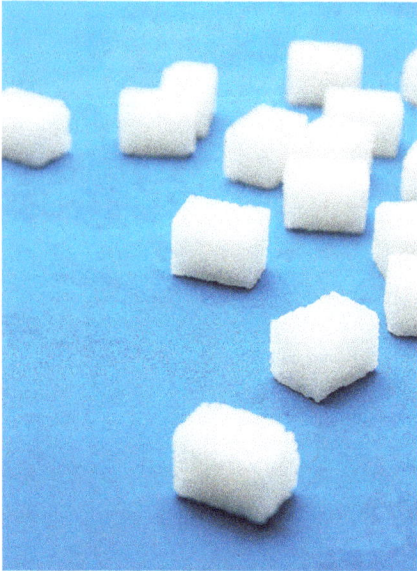

MEDIUMS FOR INTERNAL USE

Some of the following mediums may be used for the oral route: sugar cubes, honey, gelatin capsules, bread, rice flour capsules, dried powdered herb capsules, herbal tinctures, neutral tablets, milk, fatty oil capsules, charcoal, tinctures, alcohol, and syrups.

Gelatin Capsules

Gel capsules with fractionated coconut or olive oil are an optimum way to ingest harsh essential oils such as Cinnamon or Thyme. Such oils can be used for certain nervous system imbalances such as stress, insomnia, and anxiety.

Neutral Tablet

Neutral tablets are another widely used method for essential oils. They dissolve quickly and are absorbed in the mucosa of the mouth. For safety, ensure the tablet has completely absorbed the essential oils before swallowing it. You can swallow the tablet once it has dried.

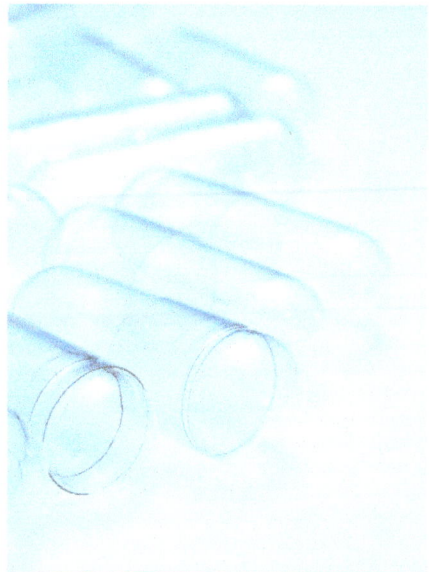

Mixing Essential Oils in Water

To emulsify the essential oils in the water, two products help make them more soluble: Solubol and Dispera. These are recommended to reduce throat irritation and digestive issues.

Solubol is a natural, non-alcoholic dispersant that quickly disperses essential oils into the water. Blend one part of essential oil with four parts of Solubol. Shake well. Add 3-4 drops to a glass of water or juice. This is also an excellent way to use essential oils in the bath.

Dispera is similar to Solubol but contains a 70% alcohol solution. Dispera also aids the absorption of essential oils by the digestive tract. Combine 80-90% Dispera with 20-10% essential oil and place one to two drops in a glass of water.

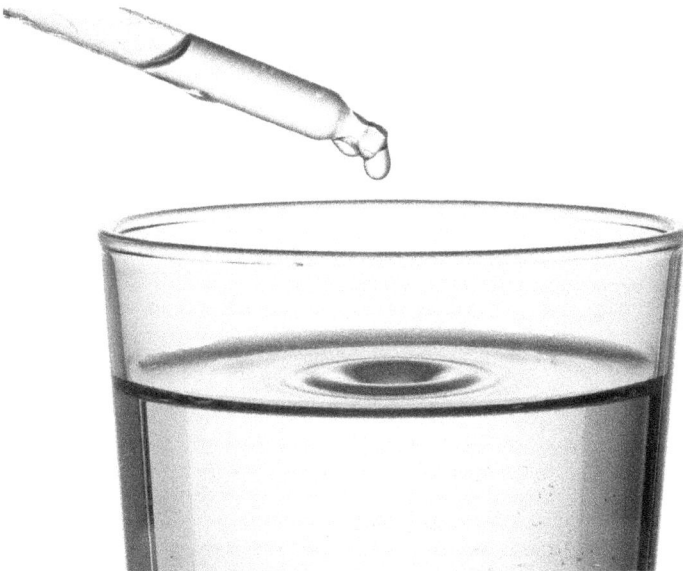

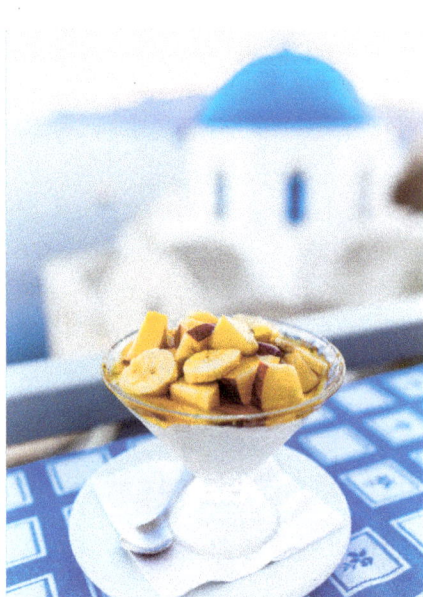

When Should You Take Essential Oils Internally?

Essential oils should typically be taken before a meal. Another option, especially when taking strong combinations (like Thyme and Cinnamon), is to take it halfway through a meal to not upset or irritate the stomach lining.

The Sublingual Route

The word "sublingual" refers to applications placed under the tongue. Essential oils are administered by placing one drop of essential oil under the tongue or one or two drops on a neutral tablet and placing the tablet under the tongue to dissolve.

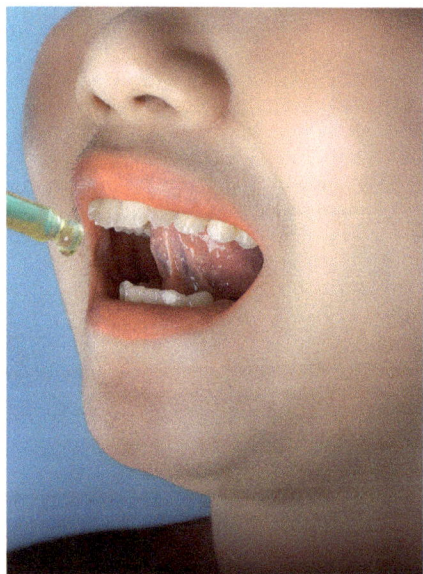

This method speeds the absorption of the molecules into the bloodstream and avoids the effect of hepatic first-pass metabolism and the gastrointestinal tract. It is most readily absorbed in this manner.

The reticulated vein underneath the tongue absorbs the essential oil components. It then transports them from the tiny facial veins to the larger jugular and brachiocephalic veins. The sublingual route is recommended for acute insomnia or acute anxiety.

Advantages of sublingual dosing:

- Fast-acting (peak levels reached in 10-15 minutes)
- Easy to self-administer
- Bypasses extensive hepatic first-pass metabolic process
- Sublingual dosing does not require swallowing
- The absorption rate is 3-10 times greater than through the oral route

> *Sublingual dosing does not require swallowing and its absorption rate is 3-10 times greater than through the oral route.*

Dosage

Sublingual dosage: 6 drops of essential per day maximum for adults with 1-3 drops per dose of non-irritating essential oils.

For adults: 1-2 drops 3-4 times/day
For adolescents: 2 drops 2 times/day
For children over seven years old: 1 drop 2 times/day

When taking sublingual drops, it is recommended to use an eye dropper and bring it in front of a mirror to be sure the application gets under the tongue. You may also use it on a neutral tablet as well.

Buccal dosage: for mouth conditions, place one drop of essential oil in the mouth between the upper and lower gums and cheek area. This can also be placed on neutral tablets.

When to use: The best time to take sublingual essential oils is before eating.

Which essential oils should you use for sublingual use?

You should use only non-irritating essential oils such as Lavender, Coriander, Lemon, etc. The only downside to this is possibly an unpleasant taste based on the flavor of the oils.

How Long Should You Use Essential Oils?

It is recommended to continue essential oil therapy for a few days or more following relief of symptoms to ensure complete healing occurs. A general rule of thumb in aromatherapy is that for every year you have suffered from a chronic condition, it could take one month of therapy to correct the condition. For acute conditions, if you do not obtain results within an hour or so, try a different essential oil or method of application. Everyone responds differently, and you may need to use more or less essential oil, depending on how your body reacts.

Rotate Your Oils

It is recommended to limit the use of the same oil or essential oil blend to twenty-one days and then take a week's break. Rotating your blends and using different oils or blends are also recommended.

This is recommended for two reasons. First, this reduces the possibility of sensitization to the essential oil or blend you are using. Secondly, this also reduces the chance of your body developing resistance or becoming acclimated to the effectiveness of the essential oils you are using. In other words, the essential oil blend may no longer work or provide the same positive benefits it once did.

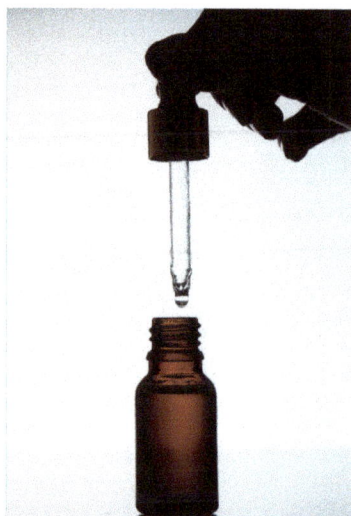

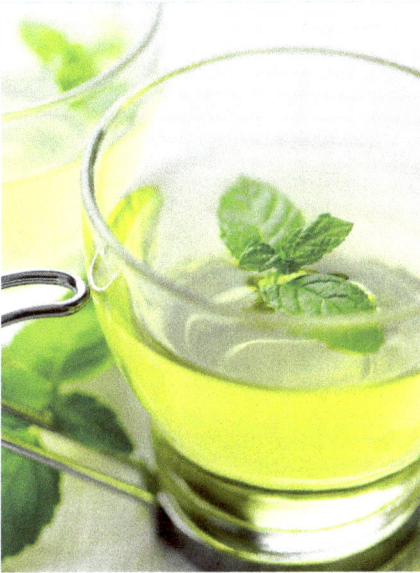

Cup of Tea

A way to calm down and de-stress is to drink a cup of warm or hot tea. Make sure your tea is not caffeinated, as stimulants can keep you awake. Add a drop or two of Bergamot or Roman Chamomile essential oil to your cup of tea for extra flavor and to help you relax. For safety, ensure any oil you add to your tea has been approved for internal use and is safe for food and drinks.

Pillow Spray

Invest in a comfortable pillow. Your pillow needs will differ depending on your sleeping habits (such as if you sleep on your side, back, or stomach). Another way to enjoy the benefits of essential oils is by applying them to your pillows and bedding to promote better sleep quality. Combine a few ounces of water and a few drops of essential oils in a spray bottle and spritz your pillows and bedding. When you lay down with your head on the pillows, you will be surrounded

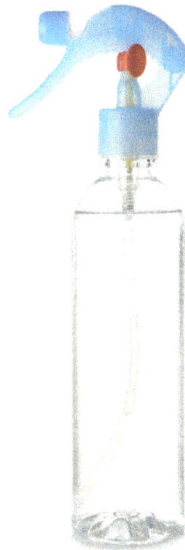

by essential oils' relaxing, comforting aroma.

Soak Away

Incorporating a Lavender milk bath into your bedtime routine can be very beneficial. Lavender milk will nourish your skin while you relax and take time for yourself. Or, adding a few drops of essential oils to a warm bath will help you calm down and comfort the body and mind before bed. Not only will a warm bath help soothe the body after a long day, but the essential oils will provide aromatic benefits to help you sleep better and wake fully rested. You can also add a few drops of oils to some Epsom salts and place them in the bottom of the bathtub. If you are a person who prefers showers to baths, you can use essential oils in the shower to help relax the mind and body before sleep. Sprinkle a few drops of a calming essential oil on the shower floor to allow the steam to disperse the aroma throughout the room. Remember to place the drops away from the water path so that your oils don't get washed down the drain immediately.

Apply Lotion with Oils

For topical applications, add a few drops of a soothing essential oil to your body lotion and apply it to the body after showering. You will smell the aroma as you begin to relax. Essential oils such as Clary Sage, Lavender, Roman Chamomile, and Ylang Ylang are calming oils that promote relaxation while nourishing the skin.

Diffuse

Turn on your essential oil diffuser while working, cleaning your home, or preparing for bed. That way, you get the benefits

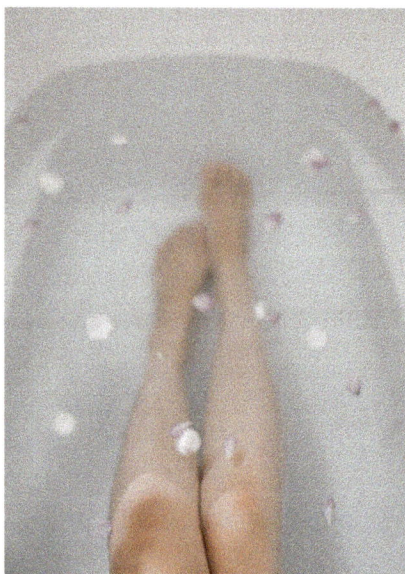

of the calming aroma as you continue to work through your to-do list. Use an oil diffuser with a timer to extend the scent lingering in the bedroom when getting ready for bed, helping you sleep peacefully through the night.

Aroma Neck Wrap

Another great way to use essential oils is with a heating pad or neck wrap to warm and relax the body. It is easy to prepare and takes only a few minutes. You simply add a few drops of essential oil to the outside fabric of a heating pad and place it around the neck or on the back for soothing warmth.

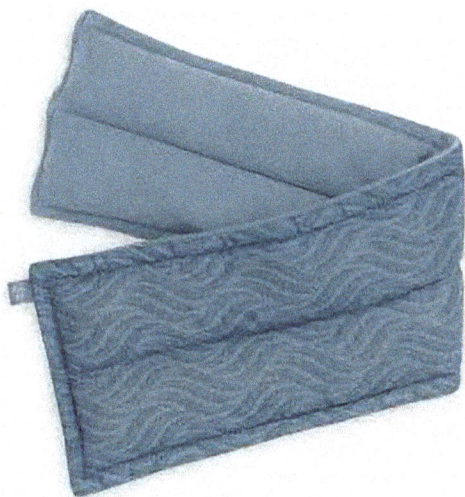

Moist Heating Pad

Here is an easy DIY non-electric heating pad that is perfect to use with essential oils. Moisten a small washcloth with water, then heat in the microwave until steamy. Remove from the microwave and add several drops of your favorite relaxing essential oil to the cloth. Place in a plastic Ziploc bag and open it slightly for the aroma to escape. Wrap a hand towel around it to retain the heat. Place it where you need it most, such as on the back of your neck or over your forehead. This method works well for children as well. Remember, some essential oils can be potent and must be diluted when used around children.

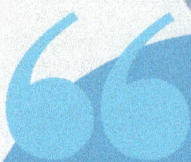

Rotating your blends and using different oils is recommended to reduce the possibility of sensitization to the essential oil or blend you are using.

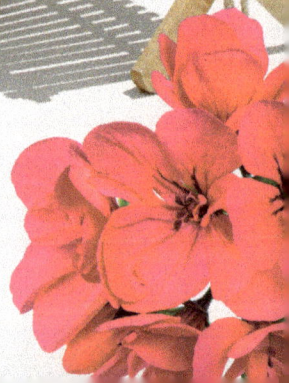

14/
CREATING BLENDS
FOR ANXIETY

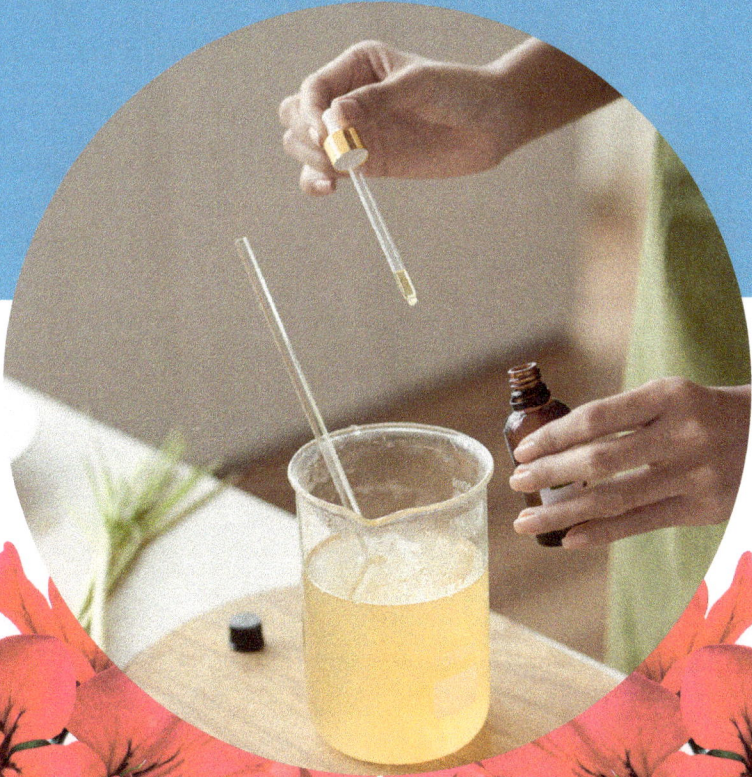

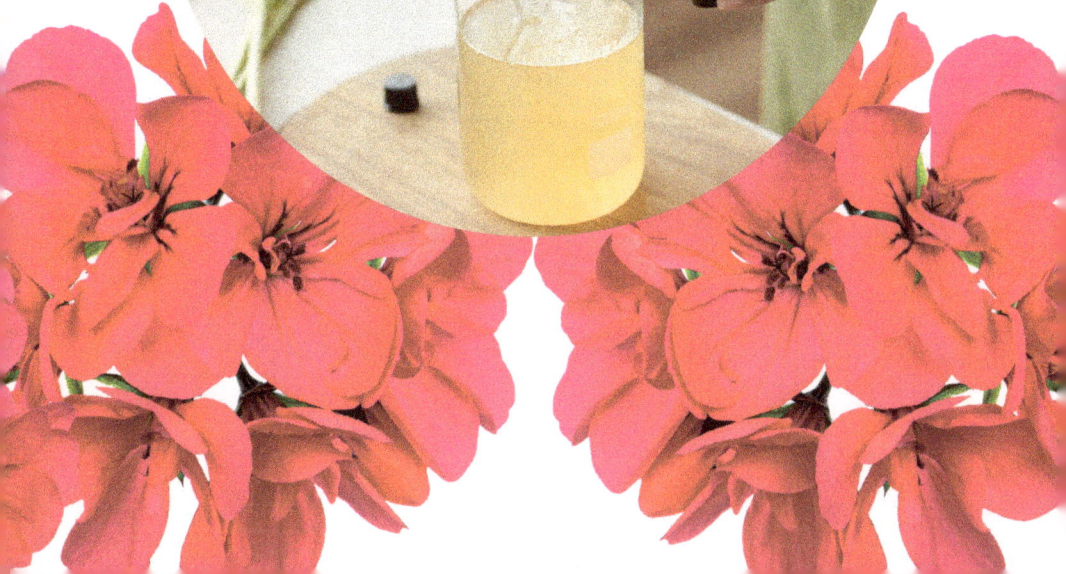

Coming up with your essential oil blend for anxiety is easy when you follow the blend-by-note technique. Your essential oil blend will contain one or more oils from these categories: Base note, Middle note, and Top note (see chart). Some apothecaries recommend using a fourth note, a fixative, or a bridge note such as Lavender, Chamomile, Marjoram, or Myrrh. The bridge is what helps the other three oils meld.

Some oils made fall into more than one category. This is possible because of the many components essential oils possess and the synergy effect a blend might draw out of that oil. However, make this work to your advantage when creating your therapeutic blends. For instance, there may come a time when you have several middle-note essential oils on hand to choose from but no top notes for your condition. In this case, you could use an essential oil that may be a top note and middle note as your top note and choose a different oil as your middle note. Follow this guide when orchestrating your blends, and let your nose have the final say.

Often vitamin E oil is used for topical blends. The following chart contains essential oils known to be beneficial for anxiousness. Each essential oil is listed by its common name and note classification: Top, Middle, and Base.

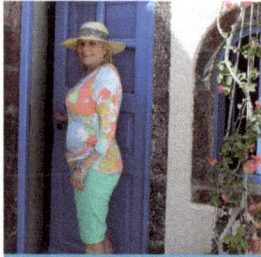

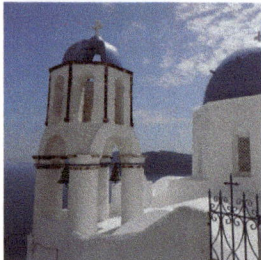

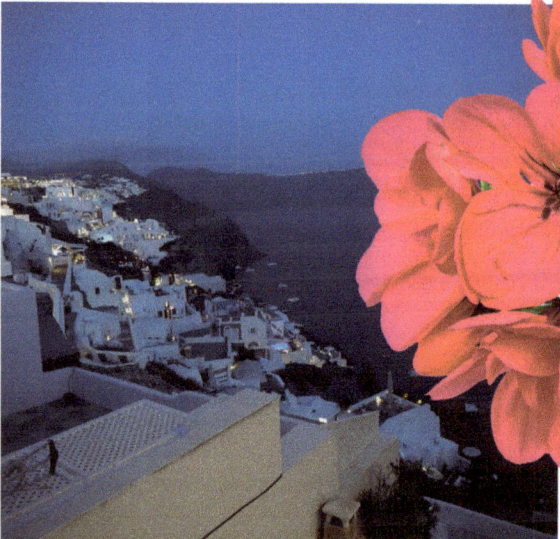

OILS FOR ANXIETY

TOP	MIDDLE	BASE
Basil	Balsam Fir	Cedarwood
Bergamot	Blue Tansy	Cistus
Lavandin	Clary Sage	Copaiba
Lavender	Coriander	Frankincense
Lemon Verbana	Fennel	Spikenard
Lime	German Chamomile	Black Spruce
Lemon Balm	Marjoram	Turmeric
Neroli	Nutmeg	Vetiver
Orange	Palmarosa	Ylang Ylang
Petitgrain	Palo Santo	
Pine	Ravensara	
Tangerine	Ravintsara	
	Roman Chamomile	
	Spearmint	

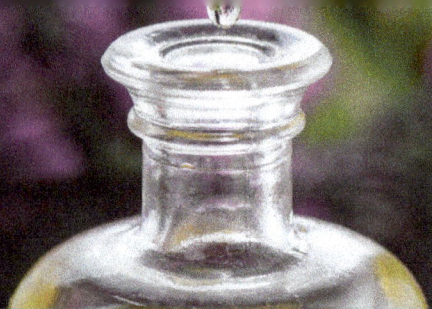

BLENDING BY NOTE

TOP NOTES

Top Notes are oils that have a light, fresh aroma. It is the first scent you smell after applying a blend to the skin. Although they quickly evaporate, the top note gives us our first impression of a blend. Familiar top notes include Lemon, Bergamot, Orange, Lime, and other citrus oils. Most top notes are made up chemically of aldehydes and esters, which are generally found in oils from fruits, flowers, and leaves.

For Therapeutic Blending: Use 3 to 15 drops of a top note per 30 ml (or one ounce) carrier.

MIDDLE NOTES

Middle Notes, also referred to as heart notes, are usually the inspiration for an aromatic blend and include floral scents such as Roman Chamomile, Lavender, or Neroli. It is generally considered the heart of the blend as it often covers any unpleasant odors that may come from the base notes. Essential oils classified as middle notes are sometimes referred to as enhancers, equalizers, or balancers. Chemically, these are monoterpene alcohols found primarily in herbs and leaves. Examples of essential oil middle notes include Lavender, Roman Chamomile, Cypress,

Geranium, Juniper Berry, Rosemary, and Peppermint. Middle notes are what we smell when the scent from the top notes fades. This scent often evaporates after 15 seconds. The middle note can last 2-4 hours in the body, and the "heart" of the blend can play on the emotions. Middle notes are often found in flowers, leaves, and needles. They also bring together the top and base notes as a "synergy" in a blend.

For Therapeutic Blending: Use 2 to 10 drops of a middle note per 30 ml (or one ounce) carrier.

BASE NOTES

Base Notes, usually the backbone and foundation of the blend, are what the users will remember most about a particular fragrance. The scent of base notes will last the longest in the air and are what you smell after about 30 seconds of applying it to your skin. The base note is added to the mixture first. Examples of essential oil base notes include Vanilla, Sandalwood, Patchouli, Frankincense, Cinnamon, or other earthy and woodsy scents. Typically, a therapeutic blend has only one base note oil as it will stay the longest on the skin and can last up to 72 hours in the body. Aromatic blends can have one or more base oils to add character. Chemically speaking, base notes are made up of sesquiterpenes or diterpenes and are mainly found in roots, gums, and resins. Though therapeutic blends typically contain one base note while aromatic blends may contain more than one, for any blend to be successful, it must have a combination of all three notes.

For Therapeutic Blending: Use 1 to 5 drops of a base note per 30 ml (or one ounce) carrier.

When making an essential oil blend for anxiety, mix the extracts in order, starting with the base note, then the middle note, and finally the top note. This ensures your blend will create an aroma known as a "bouquet" by staying in tune with odor intensity and finding notes that strike a chord and harmonize well together in therapeutic properties. Remember, for every base note drop, you add two drops of the middle note and three drops of the top note. This will ensure that your blend is well-rounded, has all three notes, and is chemically balanced between monoterpenes, sesquiterpenes, and phenols.

Structure of Aroma

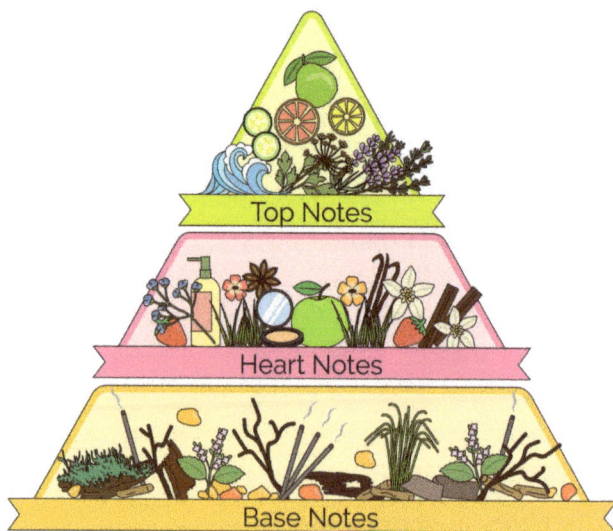

Top Notes

Heart Notes

Base Notes

MAKING YOUR FIRST ANXIETY BLEND

Now that you have learned how many drops of each note to use in your essential oil blend and have checked the precautions, it's time to start blending.

1. Gather all the necessary equipment: bottles, pipettes, essential oils, paper towels, labels, vials, and containers.

2. Ensure the counter space is clean, and your area is well-ventilated. You may want to put down wax paper (or a paper towel) to prevent any damage to the countertop from accidental spills. This will also make cleaning up much more manageable.

3. If you are using essential oils that are new to you, place one drop of the oil on a test strip (or small piece of paper) and wave it under your nose. Inhale the fragrance. If this fragrance is not what you had in mind, choose another oil and test it again. You will want to do this with each oil until you have settled on the ones you want to use for your blend. It is a good idea to have a can of coffee grounds to smell after each fragrance to clear your palette.

4. Once you have chosen the three oils for your blend, wave all three test strips fanned out beneath your nose and see if you like them. Remember that if you despise the scent, you may hesitate to use it regularly.

5. Check the safety precautions for the essential oils you have chosen to ensure there aren't any contradictions. Always consider any other health conditions, such as epilepsy or

medications, that may cause an adverse effect. Safety precautions must always be considered for the method you choose in their usage and for the person you are formulating the blend for.

6. Choose a new, clean bottle to use. Using a pipette, extract each essential oil into the bulb to place in your bottle. You may need to squeeze more than once to get the desired amount. Remember to use a separate pipette or glass eye dropper for each oil used. Add your base note essential oil first, one drop at a time. This is typically the most viscious or thickest oil. Next, add the middle note essential oil, followed by the top note essential oil. Use only the exact number of drops your recipe calls for. One drop of too many can alter the results. Replace the cap on the bottle and shake to mix oils.

7. Add your essential oil blend to a carrier oil (lotion, gel, sea salts, etc.) and blend well to distribute the oils. What you use as your carrier and how much to add will depend on which application method (Massage Blend, Bath Blend, Room Spray, etc.) you choose.

TIP: Always leave ½ inch of headspace at the top of your bottle allowing your pure essential oil blend to breathe and expand.

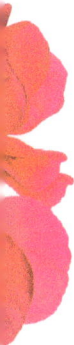

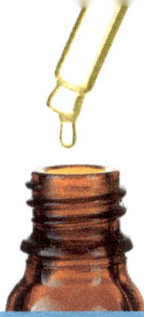

DILUTION RATE FOR YOUR BLENDS

When creating an essential oil blend for anxiety, you will need to consider the amount of carrier oil to use for dilution. Be sure to dilute correctly to ensure your blend is safe and doesn't waste your precious essential oil.

The following dilution rate chart shows you the amount of pure therapeutic essential oil to use with your carrier oil. Use a measuring spoon to add the carrier oil and a dropper to add your essential oils.

Most essential oils should be diluted for topical applications, using a 1-3% concentration of essential oils (in some cases, 5-10%). This means 6-24 drops of essential oil will be used per ounce of carrier. Therapeutic massage blends will contain between 1%-5% essential oils.

For example, adding two to three drops of pure essential oil will need diluting by adding about a teaspoon of carrier oil. For children or senior citizens, cut this amount in half.

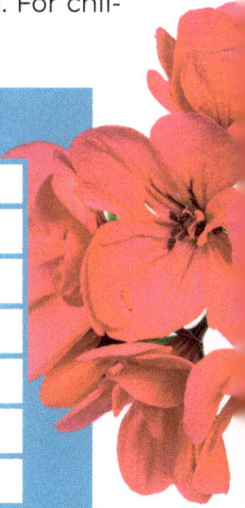

SIMPLE EVERYDAY DILUTION CHART

ESSENTIAL OIL	TO	CARRIER OIL
1 drop		¼ teaspoon
2-5 drops		1 teaspoon
4-10 drops		2 teaspoons
6-15 drops		1 Tablespoon
8-20 drops		4 teaspoons
12-30 drops		2 Tablespoons

EQUIPMENT USED FOR CREATING ANXIETY BLENDS

Before getting started, you will want to gather your supplies, such as bottles, droppers, and containers. Below is a list of the necessary tools you will need to have on hand:

Glass Bottles, preferably dark, in 5ml, 10ml, and 15ml sizes with orifice reducers (plastic dropper), can be used to make topical essential oil blends.

Glass Spray Bottles are great for making room sprays, facial spritzers, or cleaning solutions. You will find these in sizes of one-ounce, two-ounce, four-ounce, eight-ounce, and sixteen-ounce.

Small Glass Tubs are perfect for bath salts, facial creams, salves, scrubs, or other bath blends. These come in various shapes and sizes, from two-ounce to eight-ounce.

Pocket Diffusers are perfect as "personal inhalers" to carry in a pocket or purse with your favorite blend. They come with a cotton wick that saturates the essential oil inside the chamber. These are terrific for taking to work or school!

Waterproof Labels will prevent ink from running. Be sure to name each product and add the date you made the product. You will need waterproof labels in all shapes and sizes.

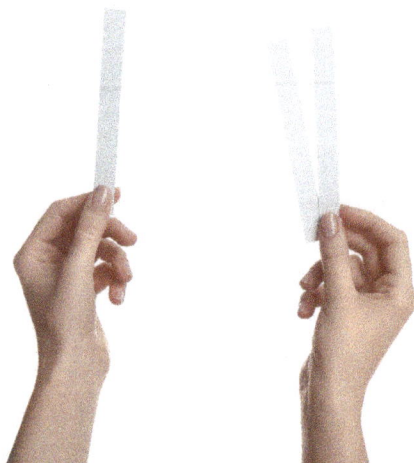

15 / ESSENTIAL OIL RECIPES FOR ANXIETY

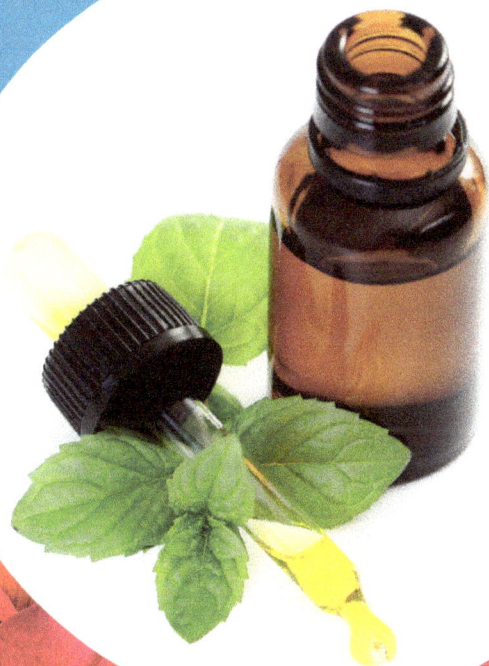

BASIC MASSAGE OIL BLEND

Here is an easy-to-follow basic recipe for making a massage blend! You get to decide which essential oils to use depending on the type of massage and the effect you are looking to achieve.

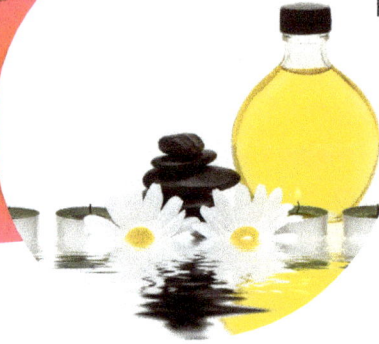

What You Will Need:

1-ounce (30 ml) Carrier Oil, Lotion, or Gel
9-15 drops Top Note essential oil
6-10 drops Middle Note essential oil
3-5 drops Base Note essential oil
Glass Bottle

What To Do:

1. Pour your carrier oil, lotion, or gel into a clean bottle.
2. Add your essential oils one drop at a time, starting with your base note, the middle note, and then the top note.
3. Shake well to mix oils and carrier.
4. Add a label with the name, ingredients, and date created.
5. Use it two to three times a day.

BASIC BATH SALTS BLEND

You can use Dead Sea, Himalayan, or Epsom salts for this basic bath salts recipe. Soak in a bath with this incredible blend to soothe the day's stress. Your bath salts can be made in advance and stored in a pretty container for convenience.

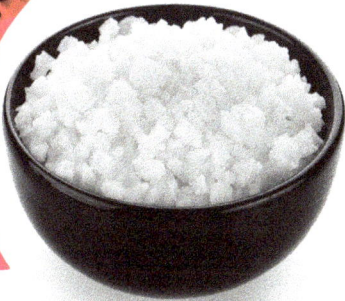

What You Will Need:

2 cups Epsom Salts
1 cup Sea Salts
1 cup Baking Soda
30 drops Top Note essential oil
20 drops Middle Note essential oil
10 drops Base Note essential oil
Wide Mouth Jar or Container

What To Do:

1. Add essential oils together in a container. Stir to mix.
2. Add sea salts and mix well to saturate the salts with the oils thoroughly.
3. Add bath salts and swish in the tub to mix thoroughly in a running bath.

Tip: Check precautions for oils that may cause skin sensitivity. It is not recommended for children.

BASIC BATH OIL BLEND

After a long day, soaking in a warm bath with a relaxing essential oil blend can be a delightful treat. Not only does it help take the edge off tense muscles, but it also ensures a better night's sleep.

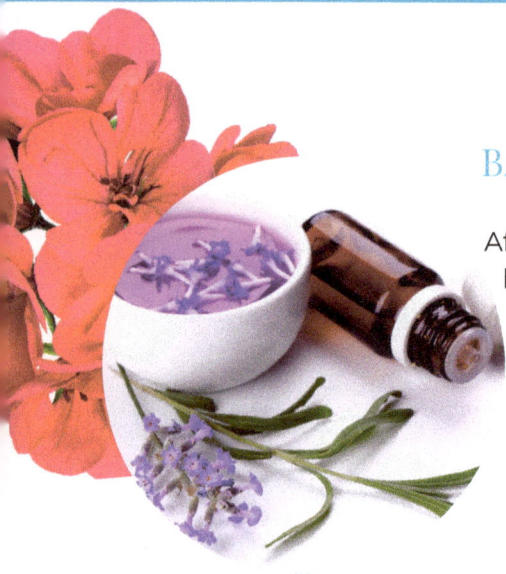

What You Will Need:

1 cup Almond oil or Coconut oil
30 drops Top Note essential oil
20 drops Middle Note essential oil
10 drops Base Note essential oil
Corked container
Crystal beads, dried flowers, tiny seashells, etc. (Optional)

What To Do:

1. Pour the carrier oil through a funnel into the corked container, leaving about an inch at the top.
2. Add essential oils to the container. Stir well to mix.
3. Cork the container and agitate the bottle gently.
4. Let it sit for 2-3 days before use. Add decor to your bottle.
5. For use, pour ½ – 1 teaspoon into the palm of your hand and gently massage into the body after a bath.

BASIC PERSONAL INHALER BLEND

Filling a new personal nasal inhaler with your essential oil blend is an effective way to experience the therapeutic power of essential oils. Inhalers are also great for many emotions, including anxiety and restlessness. They are small enough to carry in a pocket or purse and have on hand for immediate relief. Add 15-18 drops of your essential oil blend to your inhaler.

What You Will Need:

9 drops Top Note essential oil
6 drops Middle Note essential oil
3 drops Base Note essential oil
Glass Dropper
Small Plastic Inhaler

What To Do:

1. In a container, mix essential oils. Stir well to mix.
2. Use a glass or disposal dropper to fill the nasal inhaler.
3. Carry and take a whiff as needed.

BASIC CAPSULE BLEND

Here is a simple recipe for making an essential oil capsule. It is one of the best ways to take essential oils internally and bypass unpleasant tastes. You can use 1-2 drops of essential oil per capsule (depending on size).

What You Will Need:

1-2 drops Essential Oil* (20%)
Carrier Oil (80%)
Empty capsule

What To Do:

1. Separate the two parts of the capsule. Remove the top half (wider cap). You will only be filling the bottom half.
2. Add essential oil directly into the capsule, one drop at a time, using a glass dropper. This needs to be done carefully; do not add too many drops or drip oil on the side of the capsule, which will make it sticky.
3. Fill the remaining space with olive, coconut, pomegranate, etc.
4. Take the capsule immediately after filling it. These capsules will begin to dissolve right after filling them.
5. Take one capsule once in the morning and once in the evening or as prescribed by your healthcare provider.

*Only use essential oils that are safe to ingest.

BASIC BODY LOTION BLEND

Do you want to try a good body lotion recipe? Why not make your own by following these simple instructions?

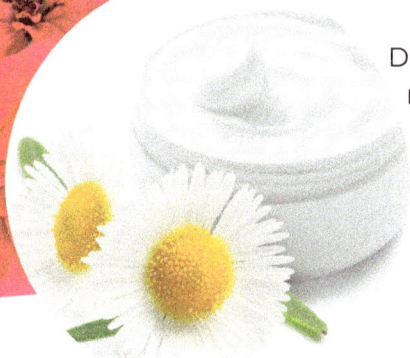

What You Will Need:

4 ounces Unscented Lotion, Hydrosol, or Carrier oil
18 drops Top Note essential oil
12 drops Middle Note essential oil
6 drops Base Note essential oil
Glass Bottle or container

What To Do:

1. Add carrier oil to the container.
2. Add essential oils, starting with your base note essential oil first, then the middle note, and finally the top note essential oil.
3. Recap and shake well to mix.
4. Use it two to three times a day.

BASIC ROLL-ON BLEND

This basic recipe can be used to create a roll-on bottle applicator for your essential oil blend, depending on the oils you have on hand. Keep track of what you add or change, so you'll know how to make your favorite blends later.

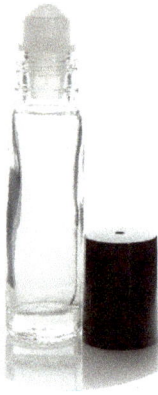

What You Will Need:

½ ounce Jojoba oil
9 drops Top Note essential oil
6 drops Middle Note essential oil
3 drops Base Note essential oil
Glass Roller Bottle

What To Do:

1. Add your carrier oil, such as Jojoba, to a dark container.
2. When adding essential oils, start with the base note and then add the middle note, followed by the top note. As you add each one, check the scent to ensure it is what you want.
3. Insert the ball and apply it 2-3 times daily.

16/

OTHER BOOKS BY REBECCA PARK TOTILO

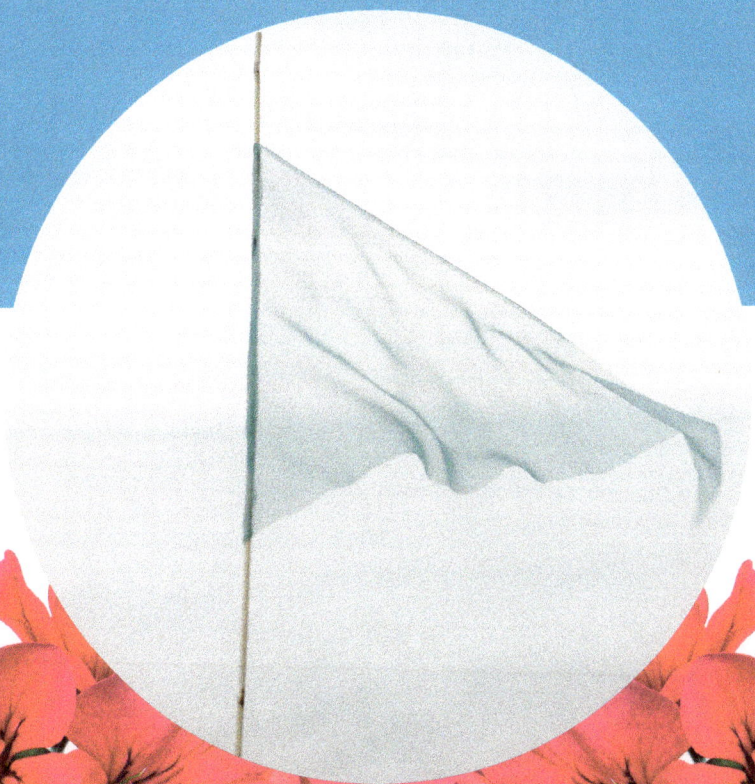

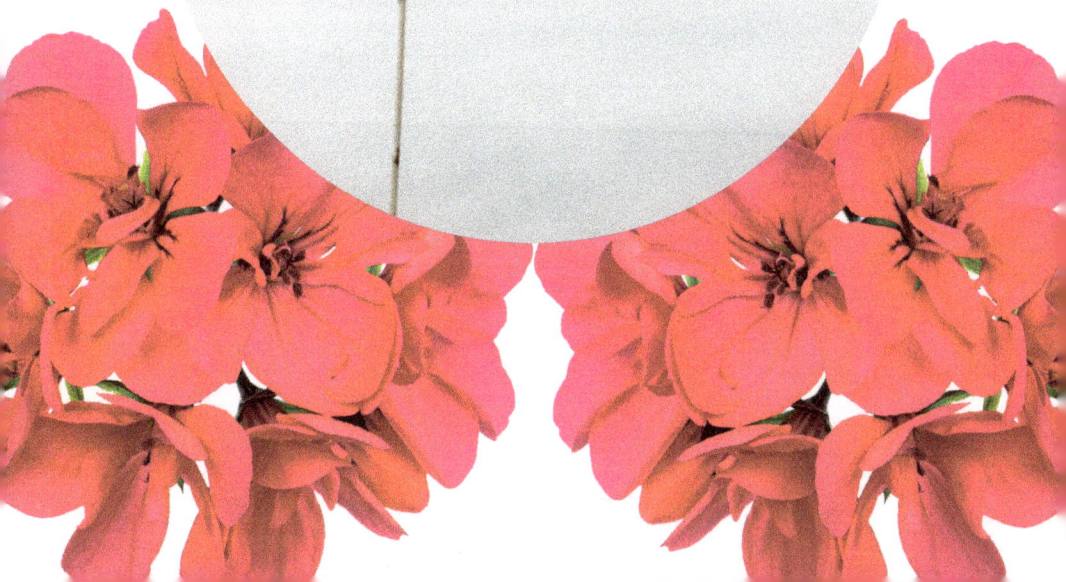

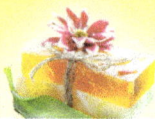

Organic Beauty With Essential Oil: Over 400+ Homemade Recipes for Natural Skin Care, Hair Care and Bath & Body Products

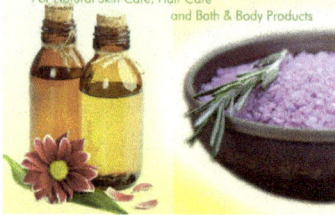

Sweep aside all those harmful chemically-based cosmetics and make your own organic bath and body products at home with the magic of potent essential oils! In this book, you'll find a luxurious array of over 400 eco-friendly recipes that call for breathtaking fragrances and soothing, rich organic ingredients satisfying you head to toe. Included you'll find helpful tips you can have the confidence knowing which essential oil to use and how much when creating your own body scrub, lip butter, or lotion bar! Discover how easy it is to make bath treats like fragrant shower gels, dreamy bubble baths, luscious creams and lotions, deep cleansing masks and facials for literally pennies using essential oils and ingredients from your kitchen.

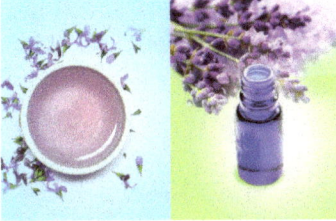

Heal With Essential Oil: Nature's Medicine Cabinet

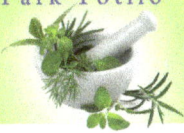

Using essential oils drawn from nature's own medicine cabinet of flowers, trees, seeds and roots, man can tap into God's healing power to heal oneself from almost any pain. Find relief from many conditions and rejuvenate the body. With over 125 recipes, this practical guide will walk you through in the most easy-to-understand form how to treat common ailments with your essential oils for everyday living. Filled with practical advice on therapeutic blending of oils and safety, a directory of the most effective oils for common ailments and easy to follow remedies chart, and prescriptive blends for aches, pains and sicknesses.

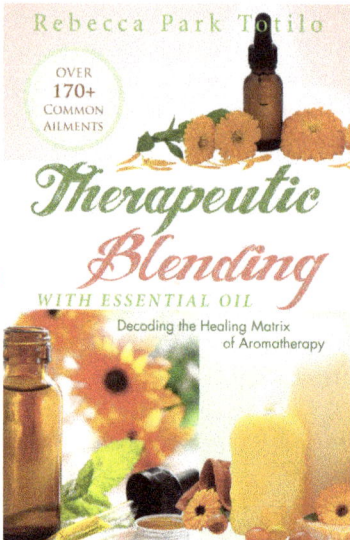

Therapeutic Blending With Essential Oil: Decoding the Healing Matrix of Aromatherapy

Therapeutic Blending With Essential Oil unlocks the healing power of essential oils and guides you through the intricate matrix of aromatherapy, with a compilation of over 170 common ailments. Discover how to properly formulate a blend for any physical or emotional symptom with easy to follow customizable recipes. Now, you can make your own massage oils, hand and body lotions, bath gels, compresses, salve ointments, smelling salts, nasal inhalers and more. This exhaustive guide takes all the guesswork out of blending oils from how many drops to include in a blend, to measuring thick oils, to how often to apply it for acute or chronic conditions. It also shows you how to create a single blend for multiple conditions. Even if you run out of oil for a favorite recipe, this book shows you how to substitute it with another oil.

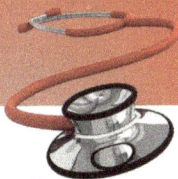

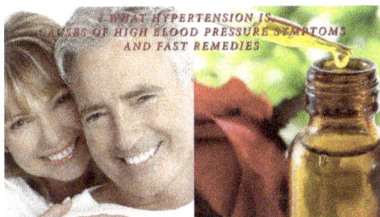

Rebecca Park Totilo

NATURAL
REMEDIES

FAST
RESULTS

HOW TO
Lower
Blood Pressure
Naturally
WITH ESSENTIAL OIL

WHAT HYPERTENSION IS,
CAUSES OF HIGH BLOOD PRESSURE SYMPTOMS
AND FAST REMEDIES

How To Lower Blood Pressure Naturally With Essential Oil: What Hypertension Is, Causes of High Pressure Symptoms and Fast Remedies

One out of three adults have it, and another one-third don't realize it. Oftentimes, it goes undetected for years. Even those who take multiple medications for it still don't have it under control. It's no secret—high blood pressure is rampant in America. High blood pressure, or hypertension, has become a household term. Between balancing meds and monitoring diets though, are the true causes—and best treatments—hidden in the shadows? In How to Lower Blood Pressure Naturally With Essential Oil, Rebecca Park Totilo sheds light on what high blood pressure is, the causes and symptoms of high blood pressure, and which essential oils regulate blood pressure and how to use essential oils as a natural, alternative method.

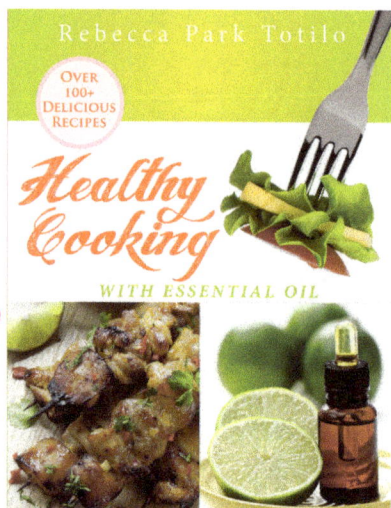

Healthy Cooking with Essential Oil

Imagine transforming an everyday dish into something extraordinary! Essential oils can enliven everything from soups, salads, to main dishes and desserts. Boasting flavor and fragrance, these intense essences can turn a dull, boring meal into something appetizing and delicious. Essential oils are fun, easy-to use and beneficial, compared to the traditional stale, dried herbs and spices found in most pantries today. Healthy food should never be thought of as mere fuel for the body, it should be enjoyed as a multi-sensory experience that brings therapeutic value as well as nourishment. For years we have limited the use of essential oils to scented candles and soaps, in the belief that they were unsafe to consume (and some are!). However, more people are realizing the value of using pure essential oils to enhance their diet. In Healthy Cooking With Essential Oil, you will learn how cooking with essential oils can open up a wealth of creative opportunities in the kitchen.

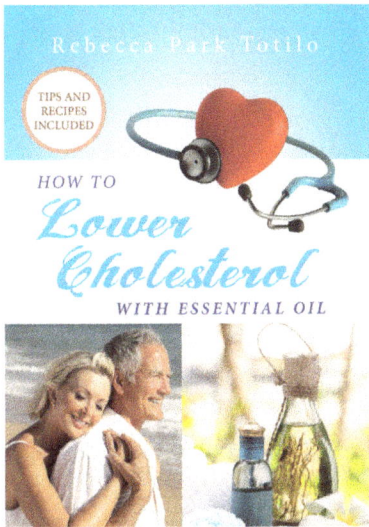

How to Lower Cholesterol with Essential Oil

Take healthy steps now to control high cholesterol and its risk factors with essential oils. People with high cholesterol have twice the risk for heart disease according to the Center for Disease Control and Prevention. What's worse, most folks aren't even aware that they have atherosclerosis until they have a heart attack or stroke. Lowering your cholesterol and triglycerides with essential oils may slow, reduce, or even stop the buildup of dangerous plaque in your arteries causing blockage of blood flow which could result in a heart attack or stroke. In this indispensable guide, author Rebecca Park Totilo presents scientific research supporting the efficacy of certain essential oils for lowering cholesterol, an extensive essential oil and carrier oil directory, natural treatments with recipes, along with easy-to-follow methods of use via inhalation, topically, and ingestion.

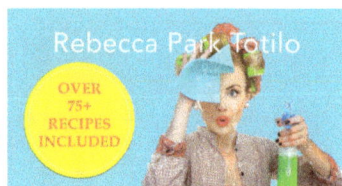

Cleaning With Essential Oil

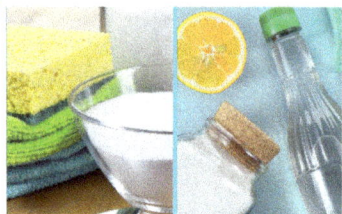

Now you can have a clean, healthy home free from harsh chemicals using a few ingredients from your pantry and essential oils! Cleaning With Essential Oil features over 75 easy-to-make recipes for every household chore, including laundry detergent, heavy-duty oven cleaner, carpet deodorizer, antibacterial wipes, stain remover, and many more!

Essential oils expert Rebecca Park Totilo guides you in choosing the best essential oils for cleaning based on their chemistry, the health benefits of cleaning with essential oils, and tips for tackling the toughest cleaning jobs from cleaning kitchen appliances to disinfecting bathrooms. The best part is she shows you how to get the entire house clean in less than an hour! Complete shopping lists for supplies and essential oils are provided, so you have everything you need for making your homemade cleaners. Now, you can turn every room into a safe and toxic-free haven for family and pets to enjoy with products like

• Simple Citrus Soft Scrub
• Stainless Steel Appliance Spray
• Lavender Hand Foaming Soap
• Peppermint Daily Shower Spray
• Minty Fresh Window & Mirror Cleaner
• Garbage Disposal Cleaning Bombs
• Lemon and Geranium Swifty Floor Wipes

In Cleaning With Essential Oil, author Rebecca Park Totilo teaches you how to make your own "green cleaners" without spending a fortune while helping save the planet! Isn't it time you ditch the chemicals and make the switch?

Aromatherapy Teacher Training With Essential Oil

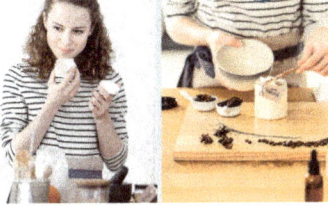

Aromatherapy Teacher Training With Essential Oil provides the essential oil enthusiast the opportunity to craft and hone effective teaching methods for facilitating essential oils classes. This informative book will help you brainstorm and develop unique and interesting aromatherapy workshops, class outlines, and, most importantly, hands-on activities that will keep your students involved and wanting more! Using Rebecca Park Totilo's personal inspirational approach to aromatherapy training, you will come away with the knowledge and confidence to lead and teach your own short workshop or aromatherapy class. Inside this instructional book, you will find:

- The Science of Teaching - Learn how to teach different learning styles, discover your teaching methodology, and develop your own personal techniques for sharing about essential oils.
- The Class - Create a lesson plan from the many themes, choose the best oils to teach, and plan your class with icebreakers, blending projects, venues, and much more.
- Teaching Aromatherapy - Discover how to introduce the safe use of essential oils with detailed step-by-step instructions on demonstrating numerous types of blending projects.
- The Business of Teaching Aromatherapy - Have confidence in knowing what to charge for your classes, develop an elevator speech, and effective marketing for your course.
- Resources - Sample outline and timelines, basic recipes, and a glossary of terms are all included.

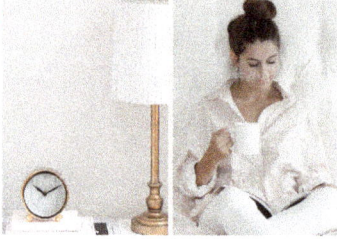

Rebecca Park Totilo

TIPS AND RECIPES INCLUDED

Sleep Better

WITH ESSENTIAL OIL

Sleep Better With Essential Oil

It can be hard to get optimal sleep in this modern age. Some people have trouble sleeping through the night because of things like a crying baby or a toddler who won't go to bed. For others, a busy work schedule and constant notifications on their phone can be distractions. And for some people, there's also the problem of having too much technology available. Social media and TV shows can be so distracting that they make it hard to get enough sleep. Even something as small and seemingly insignificant as drinking caffeine during the day or having a lumpy mattress can prevent restful sleep at night. What are we to do when distractions and outside forces steal our sleep?

Fortunately, there is hope for those struggling to get quality, consistent sleep. Hundreds of thousands of people worldwide have discovered the potent nature of essential oils to create a restful environment in their homes every night. The aroma of these oils can be combined with other healthy practices before bedtime for an even better experience. This book touches on some important aspects of sleeplessness and essential oils. Hopefully, it will answer questions you have on how to use essential oils at bedtime and create a more restful environment for getting the best sleep possible.

Rebecca Park Totilo

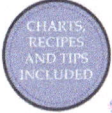

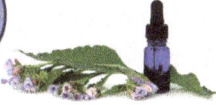

Pregnancy, Birth and Baby Care With Essential Oil

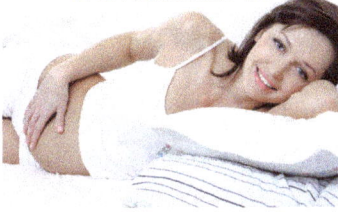

Pregnancy, Birth, and Baby Care With Essential Oil shows you how to safely use essential oils for all types of issues that arise during pregnancy, labor, and postpartum. Unlike traditional pregnancy guidebooks that follow conventional, fear-based instruction, this book offers a healthy approach to pregnancy, childbirth, and baby care, embracing a natural and safe way to use essential oils.

Full of advice and tips for a healthy pregnancy, Rebecca Park Totilo's researched-based remedies for common and troublesome symptoms guide you with the utmost care given to the health of you and your unborn child.

- Safe and Effective Essential Oils Treatments that address a range of ailments and concerns before and after the baby arrives. Details over 50 different pregnancy discomforts and challenges from morning sickness to insomnia, acne to backaches, heartburn to stretchmarks - and how aromatherapy can help.
- Numerous Charts outline specific essential oils safe for use during pregnancy, labor and delivery, nursing, and newborn care
- Detailed Profiles of 45 Essential Oils provides a comprehensive understanding of the medicinal properties, chemical makeup, and precautions of each essential oil.
- Over 100+ Essential Oils Recipes professionally formulated with step by step instructions for use in the bath, in a massage, and for diffusing around your home.

Natural Perfume With Essential Oil

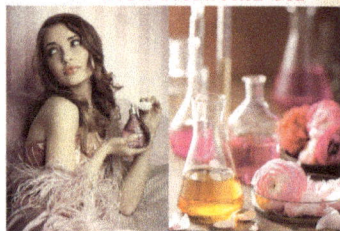

Using the same classic perfumery techniques and processes as mainstream houses, a natural perfumer can blend, dilute, age and bottle his or her own signature scent, rivaling any name brand. Perfumes, body splashes, and colognes can be healthy too when created with pure essential oils and absolutes derived from botanical ingredients harvested from the earth. Natural perfumes can be eco-friendly, unlike their lab-created synthetic counterparts whose chemicals are considered toxic environmental hazards. Now you can create natural fragrances that are subtle, giving you an aura of sweet bliss within your breathing space—only a few feet from your body. When you leave the room, your fragrance goes with you. In this guide, you will discover how to create natural Eau de parfums that develop in layers, changing gradually with the chemistry of your skin. Working in unison with your body's chemistry, your fragrance gently evolves into your own signature scent, so you smell like you, not like everybody else. Discover how to create unique fragrances unlike anything on the market that will captivate your senses.

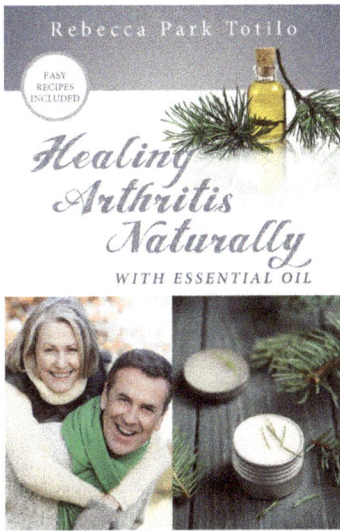

Healing Arthritis Naturally With Essential Oil

If you feel a bit like the tin man in the Wizard of Oz because your joints creak or don't move when you want them to, maybe they are asking you for oil - essential oils that is. Why live with pain or limited mobility if you don't have to? Medical research provides compelling evidence that essential oils can relieve pain and inflammation whether its due to a sports injury or arthritis, and offers the least invasive orthopedic treatment available. As the leading cause of disability in America today and the most common chronic disease to affect those over the age of 40, arthritis comes in over 100 different forms, and all share one main characteristic: joint inflammation. If you're one of the 50 million worldwide affected by arthritis, nature has provided a remedy. In this book, author Rebecca Park Totilo shares valuable information on the causes and symptoms of arthritis and how to use essential oils as a natural alternative. Discover which essential oils reduce inflammation and pain and how to formulate blends using essential oils. You will find dozens of recipes for lotions, salves, bath salts, and more in this how-to guide!

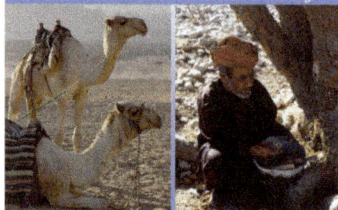

Healing In The Bible With Essential Oil

Since the creation, essential oils have been inhaled, applied to the body, and taken internally in which the benefits extended to every aspect of their being. Buried within the passages of scriptures lies a hidden treasure - possibly every man's answer to illness and disease. Now you can learn their secrets and discover how to transform your life and walk in divine health. In this book, Healing in the Bible With Essential Oil, Certified Aromatherapist Rebecca Park Totilo reveals various aspects of every fragrance mentioned in the Bible.

You will discover each essential oil:

- Rich biblical history and/or pagan roots
- Spiritual significance, symbolism, and hidden meaning
- Healing properties, including traditional uses, medicinal properties, and applications
- Scripture references, Hebrew or Greek meanings, and usage
- Rituals and recipes for making holy water, anointing oil, healing salves, and incense

Based on science and research, over 30 essential oil datasheets are included showing the breakdown of the chemical components, helping you to identify the oil's therapeutic benefits with safety information.

Stress-Free Living With Essential Oil

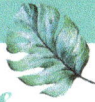

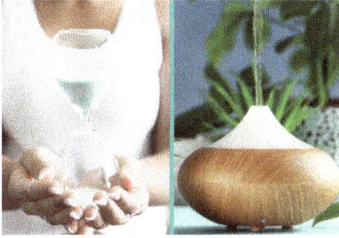

Everyone experiences stress from time to time. But when stress goes unchecked over time, it can play havoc on a person's health. Chronic stress results in a complete breakdown of the body and mental health. In Stress-Free Living With Essential Oil, author Rebecca Park Totilo offers a natural solution for handling the symptoms of stress using essential oils.

Based on scientific studies, Rebecca lists which essential oils can effectively reprogram the stress response on a chemical level in the brain and interrupt unhealthy stress responses - quickly shifting the body towards homeostasis. Discover how to live a stress-free life using essential oils. Numerous recipes and tips are included in this how-to guide!

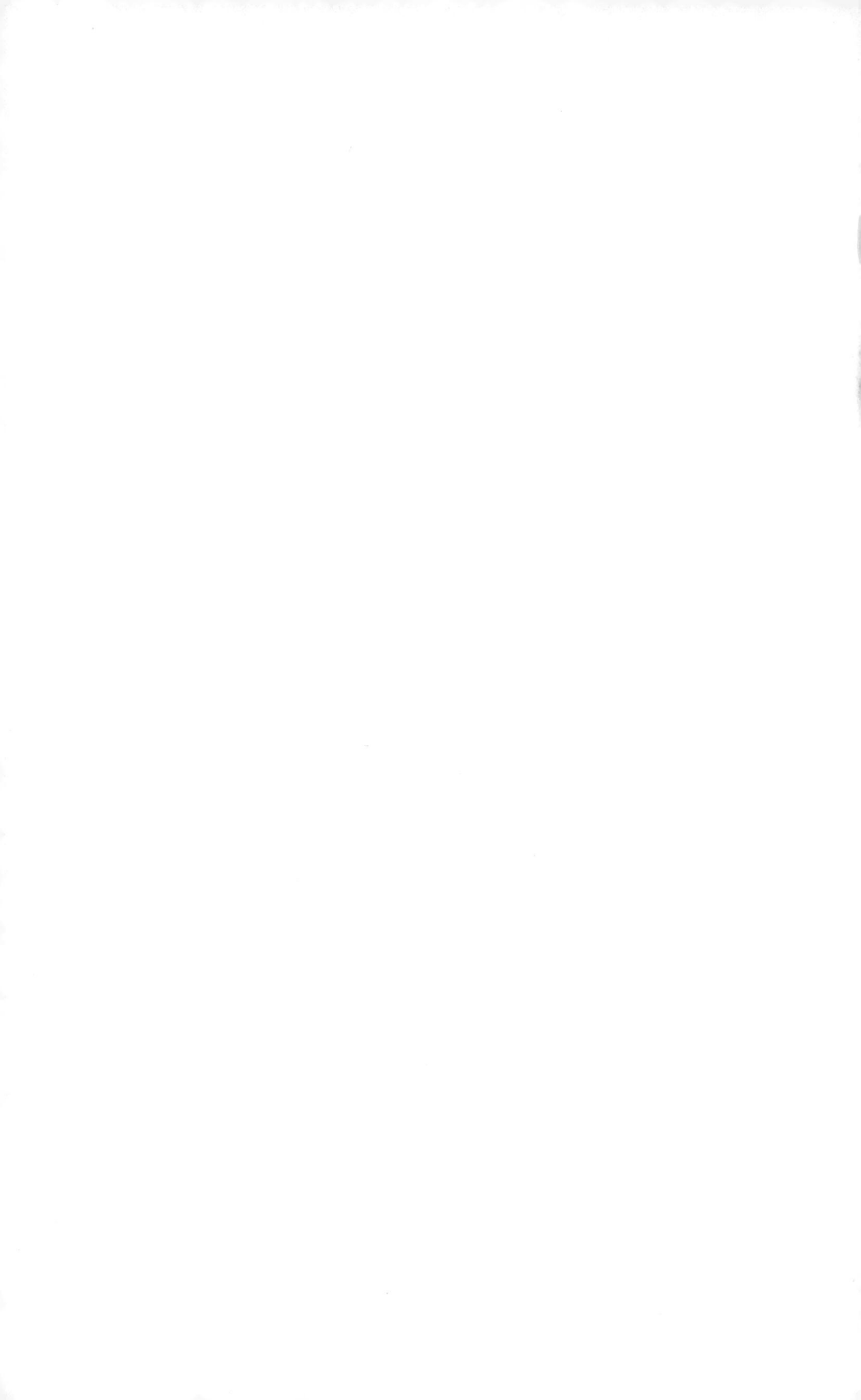

www.ingramcontent.com/pod-product-compliance
Lightning Source LLC
Chambersburg PA
CBHW050805270326
41926CB00025B/4546